SOBER FITNESS

Sober Fitness

Josh Grant

Dedication

To my brilliant and amazing wife, who somehow manages to keep me grounded while letting me chase every wild idea. Thank you for being my sounding board, my cheerleader, and one of the only people capable of reigning me in when I need it. You inspire me with your strength, dedication, and your uncanny ability to know exactly when I need snacks. You are my muse, my biggest fan, and the reason I resolve to be better every single day. I love you more than words—and *possibly* even more than coffee. (and yes, I promise to take out the trash right after this).

CONTENTS

CHAPTER 1

Introduction

I do not really remember the exact moment that the obsession of alcohol took hold of me, but I will never forget being in its grips. Every hour of every day I was either drinking or thinking about drinking. At my worst, I was drinking around the clock all day every day because I needed it to function while somehow managing to keep it hidden from the world. Without it I would not be able to think clearly, would shake uncontrollably, be unable to sleep, and have terrible nausea. I was nearly 400 pounds with sleep apnea, fatty liver, and very high blood pressure. I would binge eat because I was sad or stressed, purge in secret and feel shameful about it, then drink to oblivion to forget it all. Late at night when I had trouble sleeping—which was every night—I would drink while watching people have fun doing various things on television and wish it could be me. During the daytime, I was a bystander watching other people live. Happiness felt completely out of reach. I felt as if my life was already over and I was just waiting around to die. I did not recognize the man looking back at me in the mirror. Where was that lean handsome soldier who was once full of confidence and promise? What had happened to him?

Thanks to a God of my own understanding and a series of events, my problem with alcohol was forced into the light. I was no longer able to hide from the truth. If you are reading this and that is where you are, **know that recovery is within your reach**. I started attending recovery meetings, I got a sponsor, and I worked the twelves steps. I stumbled a little along the way, but my life has been fundamentally transformed for the better in the time since. Today, nearly 8 years sober, my life could not be more different than it was when I started this journey. I am half the weight I used to be and I can sleep at night. My sleep apnea, fatty liver, and high blood pressure are all gone. But most importantly, my family actually wants to spend time with me, I am surrounded by people who care about me, and I am living life instead of just existing.

My name is Josh Grant and I am the author of multiple books on recovery from alcoholism, addiction, and other self-destructive compulsive behaviors. If you or someone you love are still in the throes of active addiction and are looking for a book on how to get clean and sober, then I encourage you to check out some of my other books on Amazon or from my website Recovery4Life.us. I firmly believe that anyone can benefit from this book, but the aim is to help those already on the path of recovery with improving their physical and mental health. I am just a regular person sharing his own experience in the sincerest of hope that it helps someone. Please keep your own situation in mind when beginning a new exercise or diet routine and seek professional advice as appropriate for you.

For many of us, alcohol is a harmless substance enjoyed during times of celebration or an unassuming presence at a social gathering. But for others, this subtle friend reveals a darker side—a thief disguised as a friend silently stealing away our essence, health, and dreams. For those of us who lack control over it, alcohol is not just a drink. It is a cunning adversary that creeps into nearly every facet of life, leaving behind a trail of diminished health, lost opportunities, and shattered relationships. We find ourselves isolated from loved ones, trapped in cycles of self-destruction and wondering how we got there. Recovery offers the opportunity to envision a life of strength, resilience, and purpose beyond addiction.

The human body has an incredible ability to heal itself when given what it needs, particularly through proper nutrition and physical activity. During active alcoholism and addiction, many of us developed unhealthy behaviors with food, neglecting its essential role in nourishing our bodies. We may have alternated between overeating low-nutrient foods and skipping meals entirely, further weakening our physical health. This lack of balance left our bodies starved for the vitamins and minerals needed to function and repair, creating a cycle of poor health and prolonged depletion.

At the same time, our physical activity also suffered. Many of us fell into patterns of complete inactivity or sporadic, unbalanced bursts of exercise that only added strain to an already weakened body. Without regular movement, our strength, stamina and vitality deteriorated, and we felt less and less connected to our bodies. Now in recovery, we get to redesign our relationship with both food and movement, using these tools to restore balance, rebuild health in whatever way we can, and reconnect to our bodies. If we can nourish ourselves–both through what we eat and how we move–we have a platform upon which to build healing and lasting wellness.

Rebuilding health involves renewing and restoring the body's systems through a strategic combination of balanced nutrition and exercise. By nourishing ourselves with essential vitamins and minerals that it may have previously lacked, we enable our bodies to repair themselves and restore our energy levels. Regular, moderate exercise enhances this process by strengthening muscles, improving circulation, and releasing endorphins, which promote both physical well-being and mental clarity. These practices work synergistically, facilitating more effective healing and fostering an overall sense of wellness. With dedication and consistency, the body can transform, emerging stronger, healthier, and more resilient than ever before.

Good nutrition, coupled with a regular exercise plan, can help strengthen recovery from alcoholism and drug addiction by improving physical health, mental clarity and emotional resilience. But these methods are not likely enough to keep us clean and sober in and of themselves; addiction is a disease of the body, but also a spiritual and emotional sickness. The benefits of healthy living — particularly when added to a Twelve Step recovery program — go far beyond the physical and lay the groundwork for long-term sobriety. In concert, these tools treat the whole person so that by healing not just our bodies but also our minds and spirits, we greatly enhance our chances at lasting recovery.

In the following chapters, we will look at what motivates us to want change and the impact heavy alcohol use has had on our bodies to better understand where we are starting from. We will also explore a comprehensive approach to improving our physical and mental health. By addressing our physical and mental needs, we will help solidify the foundation for our lasting change and personal growth. This book will provide you guidance to support your physical self while on a recovery journey. We will learn how to set a fitness baseline and create a personalized plan, as well as how movement and meditation can bolster our physical and emotional health. You will also learn how to fuel your body with proper nutrition and the role sleep plays in optimal recovery. With a supportive environment and a focus on your overall development, you will be well-equipped to lay the groundwork for a life that encompasses not just recovery, but also strength, balance, and intention.

CHAPTER 2

Knowing Your Why

G etting sober and reclaiming your health requires discipline, re- silience, and a willingness to confront discomfort. But here's a truth that's as profound as it is simple: you cannot succeed without a clear understanding of why you're doing it. Knowing your "why" is not just a nice-to-have; it's the foundation that will keep you grounded when things get hard. Here's another truth: your "why" has to be about **you** and not about someone else. You will be able to be a better person, father, mother, son, brother, etc if you are sober—but, if your only motivation is to please a judge at a DUI hearing or keep a weary spouse from leaving you then it will be especially difficult to stay the course. You have to find within yourself the "why" you want to change. For me, it was about reconnecting with myself and being the best version of me that I could be. Others would be affected by the changes in me, but it was because I wanted to live a life of purpose that I was able to stop drinking and reclaim my health.

Every meaningful change in life starts with a reason. Perhaps you are facing some kind of crisis, or just feeling unfulfilled in life. Whatever the catalyst, your decision to stop drinking is driven by something deeper—an internal spark that should be uncovered and nurtured. When cravings strike and motivation wanes, your "why" is one of the tools you can use to keep you on track. It is fuel for your perseverance. Without it, you risk everything being temporary fixes rather than lasting commitments. On the other hand, a strong and deeply personal "why" will anchor you through challenges and temptations.

To uncover your true motivations, you need to ask yourself tough, honest questions. Why do you want to stop drinking? Perhaps alcohol has damaged your relationships, hurt your career, or taken a toll on your health. Or maybe it's about reclaiming control over your life. Why do you want to get in shape? Maybe the physical limitations of your present fitness level limits what you can do and you want to have more energy to spend with loved ones. Imagine the version of yourself who has conquered these alcohol and fitness battles. What do they feel, think, and experience daily? Be brutally honest about what happens if you continue drinking or neglect your fitness. Use this reflection as a reminder of what's at stake. Take the time to write down your thoughts. Journal them. Speak them out loud to someone you trust. The clarity you gain will be invaluable.

Sobriety is not just about abstaining from alcohol; it's also about reclaiming the parts of your life that alcohol has taken from you. Perhaps it's your health, your relationships, or your self-respect. For many, the decision to quit drinking is about rediscovering who you are beneath the layers of dependence and escapism. If your "why" is to repair your relationship with your children, visualize this reason. Imagine the moments of clarity, love, and trust you will create with them when you are fully present. Feel the pride in their eyes when they see you thriving. These images will be powerful reminders of what you're fighting for. If your "why" is rooted in health, consider how alcohol has impacted your body—from liver damage to weight gain. Picture your future self—vibrant, energetic, and free from the physical burdens of drinking. Every time you're tempted, remind yourself of the vitality you're working toward.

The decision to prioritize fitness often stems from a desire to feel better, look better, or live longer. The surface-level reasons, like wanting to fit into a smaller size or lift heavier weights, may not be enough to sustain you through the inevitable hurdles. **Dig deeper**. Why do you want to feel better? Perhaps you're tired of the sluggishness that comes from a sedentary lifestyle. Maybe you've realized that being out of shape limits your ability to participate fully in life—whether it's playing with your kids, hiking with friends, or simply climbing a flight of stairs without feeling winded. If aesthetics are a motivation, that's okay too. There's nothing wrong with wanting to look good. But pair this goal with something more meaningful. Looking good might mean feeling confident enough to pursue new opportunities, whether in your career, relationships, or personal growth.

Sobriety and health are deeply interconnected. When you stop drinking, your body begins to heal, making it easier to engage in physical activity. Conversely, regular exercise boosts your mental and emotional resilience, making it easier to stay sober. Understanding the synergy between these two goals can amplify your motivation. Imagine this scenario: You've just completed a challenging workout. Your heart is pounding, your muscles are burning, and you feel a rush of accomplishment. This moment reinforces your "why" for both fitness and sobriety. You're no longer weighed down by the toxins of alcohol, and your body is strong enough to tackle the physical demands of exercise. These victories feed into each other, creating a cycle of positive reinforcement.

Knowing your "why" is essential, but it's only the first step. To stay connected to your reasons, you need reminders that keep them front and center. Write your "why" down and place it where you'll see it daily. Break your overarching goals into smaller, manageable milestones and celebrate each achievement as a step closer to your purpose. Surround yourself with people who support your journey, whether it's a fitness class, a recovery group, or an online forum. Keep a journal of your successes, setbacks, and reflections. Periodically revisit your "why" to ensure it still resonates deeply. Your motivations may evolve over time, and that's okay.

There will be days when you want to give up. Maybe you're craving a drink after a long, stressful day. Maybe your muscles are sore, and the thought of working out feels unbearable. In these moments, return to your "why." Close your eyes and remind yourself of the life you're building. Setbacks are part of the process. Having moments of weakness doesn't erase your progress or invalidate your "why." Use these moments as opportunities to learn and grow. Resilience is not about never falling—it's about rising every time you do.

Knowing your "why" is the compass that will guide you through the challenges of sobriety and fitness. It's what will keep you moving forward when motivation fades and obstacles arise. Take the time to discover it. Write it down. Speak it out loud. Let it become an unshakable part of who you are. When you know your "why," you can endure any "how." With that knowledge, you're already on your way to a healthier, stronger, and more vibrant life.

CHAPTER 3

Understanding Impact on the Body

A couple of years before I was ready to come to terms with my alcoholism, I was at work one day and noticed my hands trembling as I tried to pour some coffee in my cup. My initial thought was that I had too much caffeine already and probably shouldn't have another cup of coffee. I went about my day. The next day when I noticed this was happening even before I had a cup of coffee, I started to wonder what might be going on but I didn't do anything about it yet. Eventually when this kept happening, I Googled my symptoms and proceeded to self-diagnose the issue. I've since figured out that Googling your symptoms is **the** fastest way to convince yourself that you are dying! I concluded at the time, that sadly I had early on-set Parkinson's Disease! I felt so sorry for myself that the only thing I could do was to have a drink. Then the most curious thing ever would happen. The trembling stopped. Why on Earth would this happen? It would be a while yet and the shaking would get much worse before I figured it out.

Understanding the effects of alcohol on the human body is a crucial first step toward making significant lifestyle changes. We often encounter information about the immediate physical consequences of alcohol consumption, but we may lack awareness of its long-term effects. This chapter offers an exploration of how alcohol use disorder can disrupt bodily functions, uncovering the often unseen changes to overall health. By examining the impact of alcohol "beneath the surface," we aim to help readers visualize the long-term outcomes of prolonged drinking more clearly. It's also likely that sober individuals will benefit from this discussion, as it allows for a comparison of experiences before and after adopting a healthier lifestyle. With a clear understanding of the material presented, those in the early stages of recovery or those seeking a healthier future can find guidance to achieve their goals, replicate positive experiences, and navigate their journey with a reliable roadmap.

In this chapter, we delve into the various health risks associated with chronic alcohol consumption, with a particular emphasis on the physical damage inflicted on vital organs, such as the liver and heart. We examine liver diseases, including cirrhosis, which is a common consequence of long-term drinking patterns. Additionally, we discuss the impact on the cardiovascular system, highlighting the increased risks of high blood pressure and heart disease that can jeopardize an individual's life.

By presenting these insights, this chapter aims to underscore the importance of proactive health management and necessary lifestyle changes. We encourage readers to reflect on their habits as they strive for sustainable wellness.

Long-term Health Risks Associated with Alcoholism

Long-term alcohol consumption can cause severe and sometimes irreversible damage to the human body. One of the most serious complications associated with chronic alcohol use is cirrhosis. Cirrhosis occurs when liver tissue becomes extensively scarred, impairing the liver's ability to function properly. This condition is alarmingly common among individuals with alcohol use disorder.

The liver is a vital organ needed to live—and is responsible for processing toxins in the blood, aiding in digestion, and storing energy. When cirrhosis develops, the liver is unable to perform these essential functions as it should, resulting in serious and potentially life-threatening complications, including liver failure and an increased risk of liver cancer.

Even moderate drinking can usher in persistent problems by inducing fatty liver disease, an abnormal condition marked by an accumulation of fat in liver cells. There are few symptoms for fatty liver, so it's dangerously easy to miss. If it is not treated, it can lead to more serious liver damage over time. Excess fat compromises liver function and can also lead to inflammation and scarring, paving the way for more serious conditions such as alcoholic hepatitis or cirrhosis. Knowing these risks underscores the need for regular medical check-ups and lifestyle modifications to support liver health.

Additionally, alcohol has detrimental effects on cardiovascular health. The risk of developing cardiovascular disease, including stroke and heart attack, significantly increases with heavy drinking. Alcohol is a known contributor to hypertension, or high blood pressure, which directly places strain on the heart and blood vessels, thereby elevating the risk of cardiac events and stroke. Furthermore, excessive alcohol consumption can lead to heart palpitations and cardiomyopathy, a condition that weakens the heart muscle and diminishes its effectiveness. These cardiovascular issues severely compromise overall heart health. Consequently, raising awareness and implementing mitigating strategies are essential for those who engage in heavy drinking.

Another concerning effect of excessive drinking is alcohol's significant contribution to weight gain and obesity. The dietary patterns of alcoholics often leads to a caloric surplus from alcohol consumption. Many alcoholic beverages are classified as having 'empty calories,' offering minimal nutritional value while consuming a substantial portion of daily caloric intake. Furthermore, alcohol has been shown to stimulate appetite while impairing self-control, which often results in poor food choices and potentially overeating. This cycle can disrupt overall metabolic balance, ultimately leading to gradual weight gain and its associated health consequences, particularly obesity.

The relationship between chronic alcohol consumption and obesity extends beyond mere caloric intake. Alcohol affects the body's ability to process nutrients, disrupting metabolism and potentially leading to insulin resistance, a significant risk factor for type 2 diabetes. Coupled with alcohol's propensity to promote weight gain, this metabolic disruption poses a serious threat to cardiovascular health and overall well-being. These factors highlight the need for better awareness on the impact of alcohol on weight management, which should be integrated into broader health maintenance strategies.

Timely intervention is essential for preventing irreversible liver damage and addressing the long-term health complications associated with chronic alcohol consumption. Early signs of liver distress—such as fatigue, discomfort in the upper right abdomen, or jaundice—should prompt an immediate visit to a physician. Routine check-ups and liver function tests are vital for detecting abnormalities at an early stage, allowing for preventive measures to be implemented before significant damage occurs. Modifying one's drinking habits or seeking professional assistance can play a pivotal role in halting or reversing potential liver damage, emphasizing the need for proactive health management.

Increasing awareness specifically about the dangers of alcohol consumption may help motivate positive lifestyle changes. And understanding the potential impacts on your liver, your heart, and your whole body can go a long way in persuading someone to reduce the number of drinks they consume. This newfound awareness can empower people to take charge of their health and start building healthier habits that contribute to their long-term well-being. By making informed choices about alcohol consumption, individuals can significantly enhance their quality of life and reduce the risk of chronic illnesses.

How Alcoholism Alters Physical Fitness

Alcohol addiction often has a negative impact on an individual's motivation to engage actively in life. Exercise is crucial for maintaining a fit and healthy body; however, alcohol use frequently depletes energy levels, making even routine tasks feel exhausting. As a result, many individuals may resort to a sedentary lifestyle, which further deteriorates their physical health. This lack of movement not only negatively affects muscle tone and cardiovascular well-being but also diminishes overall quality of life. Over time, this reduced physical activity creates a cycle that's difficult to break, where low energy perpetuates inactivity and further negatively affects mental health.

Besides promoting inactivity, alcohol interferes directly with the body's regulation of muscle maintenance and repair. Muscles should develop and replenish naturally after exercise or other physical activity. This is vital to creating strength. But alcohol disrupts protein synthesis, an essential factor in muscle building. Chronic heavy drinkers often struggle to put on the muscle they want and can ultimately experience muscle wasting over the long haul. These challenges are compounded by poor dietary choices commonly made as part of a drinking binge. This leads to decreased strength and stamina, causing reluctance to exercise.

Muscular impact aside, alcohol consumption also jeopardizes coordination and balance. Over time, the part of the brain that controls these faculties can become out of whack. This impairment heightens the risk of injuries and accidents when performing physical exercises like running or playing sports, where good coordination matters significantly. Anyone who has difficulty with balance will struggle with agile tasks and risk falling or stumbling. This not only makes it harder to maintain fitness but can also make the fear of injury more pronounced, leading to even less activity.

On the flip side, fitness routines are increasingly being incorporated into recovery journeys. Physical fitness is not only essential for rebuilding bodily strength, but it also plays a role in supporting sobriety in other ways. Exercise triggers the release of endorphins—chemicals that foster feelings of happiness and reduce the perception of pain. For individuals in recovery, these endorphins can be particularly impactful, helping to counter cravings and enhance mood. Furthermore, fitness serves as a constructive outlet, providing structure to daily life, alleviating stress, and offering a welcome respite from monotony.

Crafting a fitness routine doesn't have to be intimidating for a person in recovery from alcoholism. You can gradually rebuild confidence and capability by starting small, with activities like walking or light strength training. As strength and endurance increase, the exercises can be adapted to new comfort levels. Celebrating these baby steps helps raise self-esteem and validates progress beyond just not drinking. Discovering a life beyond just not drinking is important for long-term success.

When incorporating physical exercise, it is necessary to acknowledge individual limits. Patience is important, for the body takes time to adapt and recover from the damage of alcohol abuse. Consult professionals with knowledge in recovery from substance use when considering any new and rigorous fitness program. When used properly as part of an overall recovery plan, a proper diet and daily movement promote long-term recovery.

Additionally, joining supportive communities can provide motivation and help with accountability as well. Local groups or online communities dedicated to fitness or sobriety serve as support networks facilitating shared experiences, thus fostering an atmosphere conducive to personal growth and resilience. Also, restructuring exercise to include favorite hobbies or activities can create fun rather than something to grind, allowing for a long-term lifestyle to grow.

Weakened Immune System and Recovery Challenges

Long-term alcohol consumption can seriously compromise the immune system and may increase susceptibility to infections and disease. The immune system weakens in part because alcohol interferes with the production and activity of white blood cells, which are crucial for combating organisms that cause diseases. Also, according to the U.S. National Institute of Health, heavy alcohol use can damage bone marrow thus leading to reduced white blood cell counts, making the body susceptible to a range of infections that it might normally repel easily. With time, this reduced immunity can make people more prone to diseases such as pneumonia or tuberculosis, leading to more treatment being needed and longer recovery times than usually required.

For individuals recovering from alcoholism, gaining knowledge about and effectively managing the complex relationship between immune function and overall health is essential for both physical and mental well-being. A compromised immune system can complicate the journey to sobriety; it involves not only resisting alcohol but also addressing its detrimental effects. Therefore, enhancing immune health is integral to general healing and is vital for both short- and long-term recovery.

Alcohol's interference goes beyond simply attacking the immune system — it disrupts nutritional balance, which is crucial for the natural healing of the body. Alcohol has been shown to hinder the absorption and processing of life-saving nutrients, vitamin C, zinc, and folate. These nutrients are vital for healthy tissue repair and regeneration, functions that are inherently tied to optimal immune function. Lack of proper nutrition leaves a body incapable of its regenerative powers, and slows recovery from trauma, physical stress or even common sickness.

Furthermore, alcohol disrupts metabolism, making it challenging for individuals to maintain the energy necessary for daily activities and recovery. This metabolic imbalance raises an important question for anyone knowledgeable about basic nutrition: How can one restore their health through dietary changes? Consequently, it is essential for individuals to begin repairing their nutritional status by adopting a nutrient-dense, whole-food diet. Incorporating a variety of fruits, vegetables, lean proteins, and whole grains can help to replenish the nutrients depleted by years of neglect.

Engaging in regular physical activity brings numerous benefits—exercise activates various immune components, enhancing their surveillance capabilities and efficacy in detecting and responding to pathogens. Exercise routines don't need to be intense; moderate activities like walking, swimming, or cycling can deliver significant improvements in immune functioning. Finding enjoyable physical activities can reignite interest in movement, promote emotional well-being, and foster a healthier lifestyle overall.

Exercise is not the sole factor in enhancing immune responses; good sleep hygiene is arguably equally important. Quality sleep plays a crucial role in regulating the release of cytokines—proteins that directly combat infection and inflammation—thereby bolstering the body's defense mechanisms. Establishing a consistent sleep schedule and creating a distraction-free sleep environment further contributes to this process, as both immunity and mental clarity are essential allies in the pursuit of long-term recovery.

Beyond just exercise and sufficient rest, stress management plays a pivotal role in supporting immune system response. Chronic stress has been shown to lower immune capacity. Meditation, yoga, and deep-breathing exercises are powerful tools to alleviate stress and cultivate mindfulness. These practices enhance physical recovery efforts and promote the "one-day-at-a-time" philosophy of recovery by bringing our thoughts to the present.

Our diets also have an impact on our immune system. Incorporating antioxidant-rich foods, such as berries, nuts, and leafy green vegetables, strengthens the body's defenses. To optimize your diet, consider including foods rich in omega-3 fatty acids such as flaxseed and eggs or salmon to help reduce inflammation. Additionally, kombucha and yogurt along with other fermented foods provide probiotics that promote gut health, ultimately enhancing your immune response.

Hydration is a crucial component of any comprehensive approach to wellness that should not be overlooked. Alcohol functions as a diuretic, leading to dehydration and impairing cellular functions essential for optimal immunity. To enhance disease prevention and recovery, it is important to drink sufficient water daily. Proper hydration helps the body effectively absorb nutrients and eliminate toxins, promoting overall health.

Immune resilience is not solely determined by any single lifestyle factor; rather, it emerges from the harmonious integration of various elements that together restore the body to a state of balance. While implementing these changes requires effort, the benefits are substantial. The journey may involve important 'must-dos' and 'can-dos,' but the challenge is undeniably worthwhile. Not only does this approach prove effective, but it also fosters habits that contribute to long-term health and longevity, extending well beyond merely reversing the effects of alcohol consumption.

With the right exercise routines, people can find a greater sense of self-efficacy when it comes to getting active again — allowing them to feel in control of their own fitness journeys instead of letting fitness goals intimidate them. Exercising in a way that fits your abilities and preferences makes it more likely that you'll stick with it and helps you feel proud of what you achieve. Celebrating your achievements, big and small, fosters dedication to replacing the harmful legacy left by alcohol because every single step brings you closer to a more whole, more resilient body.

Understanding the impact of alcohol abuse goes beyond just its short-term effects; the physical consequences can have long-term ramifications for several bodily systems. In this chapter, we explored how excessive drinking affects liver function, heart health, and metabolic function. Whether it is the progression to cirrhosis or the complications of cardiovascular diseases: the pernicious effects of alcohol to undermine health itself cannot be overstated. Even moderate intake is enough for conditions like fatty liver disease and hypertension, making attention and prevention vital. Learning about these potential outcomes is important for every individual pursuing sobriety or wishing to protect their personal well-being. Regular check-ups and lifestyle changes are key and could help as we live longer lives.

The pathway to better health includes recognizing how alcohol abuse affects your physical fitness, how it impacts immune system strength, and how it will affect recovery. Identifying precursors and adding healthy practices including nutrition and exercise can change the story against alcohol's nefarious legacy. Creating circumstances in which they can make well-informed decisions and leading lifestyles to actively regain ownership in their health. Education, action, and perseverance can start to heal some of the damage endured through alcohol abuse and promote a lifestyle that embraces longevity and resilience.

CHAPTER 4

Mental Recovery—A Return to Clarity

One day while still in active alcoholism, I came home from work to a very unhappy wife and a dark house. When I say the house was dark, I do not mean that metaphysically. I mean the power had been cut off that day for non-payment. My wife had already figured out the problem and paid the bill over the phone but it would be a couple of hours before the lights were back on. To this day, I do not exactly know what happened or why I did not pay the bill on time. We had the money, and I distinctly remembered sitting down at my computer to pay bills one morning before work—with a drink of course (spoiler alert: it wasn't a morning coffee). The most disturbing part was that I didn't remember what happened next. I didn't remember paying the bill or not paying the bill. I didn't remember going to work or anything that happened the rest of that day. I didn't even realize that the day was missing from my memory until that moment when I was faced with the fact that the electricity was turned off. It seems so obvious now looking back on it, but I was utterly without explanation at the time about what had happened. I thought I was losing my mind. It was scary and depressing—so, of course I needed something to drink to calm my nerves and lift my mood. That kind of madness would unfortunately continue for a few more years before I found sobriety.

Mental recovery following addiction is a profound journey filled with opportunities for growth and change. The mind, just like the body, undergoes significant changes during and after addiction, leaving many wondering how to regain mental clarity. In this chapter, we will look at the amazing capabilities of the human brain to heal from the harms of addiction. We will explore ways to help reverse cognitive decline caused by abusing substances and highlights techniques that promote mental restoration. The chapter discusses an array of strategies, from doing cognitive work such as puzzles, brain games, and memory games to mindfulness and journaling. During this conversation readers will learn how to improve memory, attention, and, overall, mental health, and gain a deeper understanding of the resilience and adaptability of the mind.

Cognitive Improvements Post-Sobriety

Walking the road to sobriety isn't just about making physical changes—it's a mental journey too. One important part of this process is the brain's natural ability to adapt and change. When you stop drinking, this becomes especially important. Long-term alcohol use can do significant damage to your brain, leading to problems with memory, focus, and decision-making. But when you remove alcohol from your life, your brain can start to heal and rebuild itself, undoing much of the damage. This rebuilding process creates the foundation for clearer thinking and better mental function.

Beyond biological changes, actively engaging in cognitive activities plays a pivotal role in enhancing mental recovery. These activities could range from puzzles and brain games to reading literature or even learning a new skill like playing a musical instrument. Such engagements encourage the brain to forge new connections and improve existing ones, leading to clearer thinking and better focus. Participation in these tasks stimulates mental engagement and helps to maintain motivation during the recovery journey. By continuing to challenge the brain, individuals not only bolster their cognitive functions but also foster a sense of accomplishment and productivity.

Memory improvement methods can be instrumental in supporting mental recovery. One particularly effective tool is journaling. More than just a daily record of activities, journaling serves as a mental workout, strengthening the connections between neurons and providing a cognitive boost. Writing down your thoughts, experiences, and feelings helps organize information, facilitates retrieval, and encourages deep emotional processing. Additionally, journaling allows you to reflect on daily events, recognize thought and behavioral patterns, and gain insights into your emotional state. Even recording the details of everyday life can significantly enhance memory retention. Research in psychology suggests that these practices not only bolster emotional health but also offer distinct benefits that promote overall cognitive function.

As we progress in sobriety we will likely notice improvements in our attention span as well. In the absence of alcohol-induced distractions, individuals experience increased focus and productivity. The mind becomes less cluttered, allowing for better concentration on tasks at hand. This newfound attentiveness doesn't just apply to work or studies; it extends to daily interactions and decision-making processes. With fewer distractions clouding judgment, individuals are better equipped to engage in mindfulness practices. Mindfulness involves being present, paying attention to thoughts and feelings without judgment, which ensures continuous growth of mental clarity. It fosters a deeper understanding of oneself and promotes thoughtful responses rather than impulsive reactions.

A guideline worth considering is integrating engagement in cognitive activities into daily routines, especially for those newly on the path to sobriety. Developing a habit around such practices not only accelerates mental recovery but also builds resilience against potential relapses. One could start with simple exercises like crossword puzzles, gradually progressing to more complex activities like painting or learning a new language. Establishing a routine where these cognitive activities are performed regularly can create a structured environment conducive to growth and healing.

Mindful attention, bolstered by sobriety, allows individuals to savor moments that were once overshadowed by substance use. Whether it's focusing clearly on a task at work or enjoying a quiet moment with family, the ability to be fully present becomes a cherished outcome of the recovery journey. As distractions diminish, so too does the anxiety often associated with them. This reduction in stress leads to increased productivity, allowing individuals to achieve goals that seemed unattainable during periods of addiction.

The mental recovery after addiction is both meaningful and rewarding. Sobriety clears the way for sharper thinking and new opportunities. Breaking free from substances brings a fresh sense of clarity and the chance to improve how your mind works. Engaging in activities like solving puzzles, writing, and practicing mindfulness can help fill the void and strengthen your focus. This process shows just how adaptable people can be and highlights the incredible potential of the human brain once it's free from the grip of addiction.

Managing Emotional Turbulence in Recovery

Another critical characteristic of recovery from alcoholism and addiction is learning to navigate through and regulate emotions. Awareness of emotional triggers might be an important starting point on this road. Emotional triggers are either that experience or memory that elicits strong emotional response, likely connected to past circumstance. Becoming aware of these triggers enables people to pre-empt their responses and come up with coping mechanisms before they are swallowed by their impulses. For instance, if social environments where alcohol was previously consumed become a trigger for craving, acknowledgment of this fact helps in devising strategies to maintain sobriety. A journal can be an excellent tool here—a space to document situations and feelings, helping to unveil patterns over time. It is through these revelations that one finds power in understanding and controlling external and internal stimuli.

After identifying triggers, the next step is practicing healthy coping skills. Regular physical activity is well-known to enhance mood and relieve stress. Whether it's a brisk walk in the park, cycling, or engaging in structured exercise routines, endorphins—naturally uplifting chemicals in the brain—are released when we move our body. Another great method is deep breathing exercises which calm the nervous system and allow your focus to switch from stressors to that of relaxation. Picture yourself finding a quiet corner, closing your eyes, and inhaling deeply through your nose, allowing your chest and abdomen to expand before exhaling slowly. With practice, this becomes a quick escape to tranquility amid chaos.

Artistic expression should not be overlooked either. Making creative outlets such as sketching, painting, or even dancing available provides new avenues for the regulation of our emotions. These are creative forms of expression that may help convey things that are too hard to explain in words, providing release from pent-up emotions. They can also be especially helpful for people who may have difficulty articulating their thoughts or feelings, giving other pathways for expression and clarity.

In addition to these methods, mindfulness meditation and Cognitive Behavioral Therapy (CBT) provide key tactics to improve emotional regulation. Mindfulness encourages people to live in the moment, paying attention to what their thoughts and feelings are in the present without judgment. Research has proven regular meditation practice helps reduce anxiety and depression, which are both vital for emotional health. Mindfulness can be simply taking ten minutes a day to settle on your breath every morning or just considering your surroundings and what you feel without getting caught up in it.

Conversely, CBT arms people with tools that allow them to encourage and modify negative thought patterns. One of the most helpful suggestions of my sponsor was to talk to a professional therapist who utilized CBT techniques in his practice. CBT teaches individuals to understand the connections between thoughts, feelings, and behaviors, making it possible to change maladaptive thought patterns. Someone who feels their anxiety rising about attending the event could reframe it using CBT techniques, potentially lowering anxiety and improving their emotional outcome. While mindfulness nurtures presence, CBT provides practical frameworks for altering perceptions and reactions.

Building a supportive community is another cornerstone in the recovery process. It's often said that 'it takes a village,' and this holds true when navigating emotional recovery. Being surrounded by understanding peers who have walked similar paths offers comfort and motivation. Support groups or recovery meetings present opportunities to share experiences and learn from others' journeys. Within these settings, one might find solace in knowing that they are not alone, which can be incredibly empowering.

Beyond peer support, seeking professional help is also paramount. Therapists and counselors possess the training to offer guidance tailored to individual needs. They can provide insights that may not be apparent to those in recovery, helping to navigate complex emotional landscapes. Often, simply having a safe environment to voice fears and worries can lighten emotional burdens significantly.

Critical Thinking Abilities

For individuals struggling with addiction, achieving sobriety serves as a crucial foundation for developing essential problem-solving skills. Addiction often inflicts significant damage on mental health, making it necessary to undertake a comprehensive repair of cognitive function. This newfound clarity brings about a profound shift in perspective. Clearer thinking paves the way for better decision-making and sounder judgment—both of which are vital for establishing and maintaining healthier relationships.

Addiction can impair the brain's cognitive functions, impeding one's ability to reward oneself or steer away from life's challenges. The haze that clouds rational decision-making lifts in sobriety. This newfound mental clarity illuminates pathways to solid mental acuity. When people start to get their mind back, they start to cultivate better relationships with other people. These connections serve as a foundation for continued recovery, positivity and support of one another.

This progress is furthered with challenging activities that hone the analytical skills. Mental capacity stretching endeavors, like riddles, strategy games and skill development, invigorate the brain, leading to increased growth. Unlike the mad scramble of addiction, where the only thing that matters is immediate gratification, these pursuits demand patience, strategy, and foresight. Sober living teaches you to find pleasure in critical thinking and problem solving as opposed to allowing yourself to be led back to your compulsive ways.

Enhanced cognitive functions play an important role in day-to-day functioning and the quality of life overall. Sobriety helps in getting out of the bed and swinging through the entire work of the day with better focus and remembering capabilities. The simple routines that felt arduous under the fog of addiction become bearable, even rewarding. From booking personal calendars to fulfilling work obligations, all areas of life reap the rewards of refreshed brainpower.

What if you could organize a meal without missing a single ingredient, never forget an appointment and hold the other end of a conversation without losing flow? Through these banal but vital tasks a sense of normality and routine is slowly but surely reestablished, building confidence in daily exchanges. As a result, people are able to slip back into their roles in society more smoothly at work and in community and family settings.

Sobriety leads to significant cognitive improvements empowering individuals with enhanced critical thinking skills. Addiction often constrains thought patterns, leading to repetitive and narrow-minded approaches. In contrast, sobriety opens up diverse perspectives, enabling creative problem-solving and innovation. With a clear mind, individuals can break free from habitual thought loops, examining issues from multiple angles with insight and curiosity.

This empowerment is reflected in transformative ways. For example, when a sober person encounters conflict at work or home, they may actively consider various solutions instead of reverting to old coping strategies. Critical thinking inspires negotiation, compromise, and common ground, all instrumental in creating an environment that is supportive of healing and growth.

Furthermore, developing such cognitive agility has broader implications. It unlocks opportunities to pursue educational endeavors or career advancements once deemed unattainable. Whether enrolling in courses, engaging in professional development, or actively participating in constructive dialogues, critical thinking serves as a catalyst for unlocking potential previously stifled by addiction.

While exploring these advancements, it's essential to incorporate mindfulness practices to sustain attention over time. Mindfulness helps maintain focus and supports ongoing cognitive enhancement. By cultivating awareness of the present moment, individuals can redirect wandering thoughts, fortify concentration, and reinforce mental resilience.

For those seeking to harness the breadth of cognitive possibilities in sobriety, mindfulness offers simple yet profound guidelines. Techniques such as meditation, deep breathing exercises, and mindful observation of daily activities provide steady anchors. Through regular mindfulness, individuals can cultivate an environment within their minds where clarity and creativity flourish side by side.

Final Insights on Mental Recovery

Restoration of mental health after an addiction is really intentional and hard. However, with that sobriety comes many paths to a clearer mind and a more stable heart. Due to your brain's ability to rewire itself, you're returning back to a state of clarity and focus that may have been dulled or lost due to addiction. You also motivated yourself and achieved a sense of accomplishment by reading, learning new skills, and doing mental activities like puzzles and brain teasers. Journaling can be particularly beneficial, as it provides structure and aids in memory retention.

Alongside the cognitive enhancements, handling emotional roller coasters forms a key part of healing. By being aware of and anticipating emotional triggers, you can choose to respond with intention, rather than react in the moment. These healthy coping strategies, including exercise, mindfulness meditation, and creative expression, help to stabilize emotion and reduce stress. Techniques from Cognitive Behavioral Therapy provide actionable steps to change thought patterns, leading to improved emotional effects. Having a supportive community surrounding you deepens this process, providing encouragement and understanding through the process. Hence, even though sometimes it may seem that sobriety only causes you to miss out on the best part of your life, in actuality, it removes the chains of addiction and enables you to be able to heal at an emotional and cognitive level and helps you approach your life with a more resilient and purpose-driven mindset.

CHAPTER 5

Setting a Fitness Baseline

I've come to realize in the years since I quit drinking, that my biggest obstacle in life is me. If I want to hike the Grand Canyon, or become a doctor, or go skydiving, or learn another language—then, the only thing stopping me from doing it, is me. All I need is determination, belief in myself, and to put action behind a realistic plan to make those things happen. For too much of my life, I allowed fear and self-doubt to dictate what my future was or wasn't.

In recovery, my entire perspective on life has been flipped around 180 degrees and I realize that I can do just about anything I set my mind to. Of course, there are limitations to this. I'm not advocating that anyone can learn to fly by flapping their arms and just believing in themselves enough. But with the right plan and consistent action I **can** transform myself from the morbidly obese guy—who gets winded going upstairs at home—into someone capable of hiking the Grand Canyon.

The starting point of any realistic plan is an honest assessment of where you are starting from. I think of it sort of like a 4th step inventory where we made "a searching and fearless moral inventory of ourselves". In this context, it would be a thorough and honest assessment of where we are physically. The purpose of this isn't to beat ourselves up but to help establish our baseline health metrics and what our strengths and weaknesses are. Being able to identify these empower you to create an effective and safe fitness plan that suits your needs. Recognizing and acknowledging this prepares the path for a more fulfilling and sustainable process of achieving better health.

This chapter covers the basics of determining your basic fitness level. We also examine how personal variables such as prior injuries, body composition and current health status significantly influence your starting point. By analyzing what your body is capable of (and not capable of), we provide insight into how to tailor your routine in a way that works for you. In this chapter, you will also learn about strategies to monitor changes and progress over time, allowing you to make informed changes that will support ongoing growth. Furthermore, we stress the need for professional advice to safely navigate the complexities of personal fitness journeys. By the end, you'll have the information and the tools to get you started on a personalized journey to better physical and mental health.

Recognizing Physical Limitations

It is important to acknowledge that embarking on your first fitness journey or embracing sobriety after a long and challenging period requires a fresh start. This process often involves learning from the ground up, albeit through some difficult lessons. The core principle here is that when individuals understand what to expect, they can better align their goals and avoid unforeseen obstacles.

It is essential to recognize that no two bodies are the same. Factors such as body composition, past injuries, and other health conditions will influence how exercise impacts each individual. This inherent uniqueness underscores the necessity for personalized attention when developing a fitness regimen.

Much like different materials will react differently when placed under stress, fitness is not one-size-fits-all. Some people love to run, others are put off by aching joints. Such differences require a greater understanding of how everybody responds to exercise. This means that by paying attention to such different responses at the individual level, one may modify training to the individuals, leading to progression and not to frustration. Examples include an individual who has a higher ratio of fast-twitch muscle fibers, who would likely excel in short distance sprints rather than long-distance endurance, thus suggesting that, when deciding on an exercise regime, it should be tailored to one's innate capabilities.

It is also important to acknowledge the role of any physical limitations, including chronic pain or fatigue. They can be flags to potential health conditions the individual may not be aware of which may need to be addressed prior to beginning an exercise routine. Chronic knee pain, for instance, may be due to an old injury requiring rehabilitation or may indicate arthritis. Dismissing these warning signs will only cause more harm, endangering not only your physical health but preventing you from feeling incentivized and making progress.

One sensible option is to begin doing gentle movements that don't increase pain or fatigue. Yoga or swimming, for instance, can provide low-impact alternatives that strengthen and stretch without straining trouble points. Body awareness becomes paramount here; if something you do elicits discomfort or pain, it's important to modify or find alternatives. The goal should always be improving overall well-being without compromising safety.

Providing room for gradual progression is also essential. Rather than jumping full throttle into a demanding fitness schedule, incrementally increasing intensity can yield far better results and reduce the risk of injury. A structured plan that begins with shorter, less intense sessions and gradually builds up can be highly effective. It allows the body to adapt and strengthen over time, ensuring that each workout contributes positively towards fitness goals.

Consulting professionals can significantly aid in this process by offering personalized advice tailored to one's specific needs. Fitness trainers or physiotherapists can assess an individual's current state and work collaboratively to design a program that respects their limitations while fostering growth. This professional guidance ensures that workouts are conducted in a safe manner, helping to prevent any potential harm.

Monitoring changes throughout the fitness journey is another cornerstone of success. Keeping track of how the body responds to various exercises enables adjustments that maximize effectiveness while minimizing adverse effects. Documenting symptoms, energy levels, and recovery times can provide valuable insights. If cycling initially caused discomfort but seems to improve energy levels and stamina over time, this feedback can encourage continued effort in that area. Conversely, if lifting heavy weights consistently leads to painful joints, exploring lighter weight options or alternative exercises might be preferable.

The ultimate aim is to develop personalized workout strategies that respect individual constraints and enhance both safety and effectiveness. Embracing and respecting limitations does not imply settling for less; rather, it means leveraging what works best for you and building upon it. Crafting a personalized plan transforms perceived boundaries into stepping stones towards achieving greater health and fitness levels.

Consulting and Monitoring for Effective Progress

Beginning a fitness journey is often a daunting task, especially for those newly venturing out of sobriety or anyone aiming to improve their health after a long hiatus. Employing professional guidance along with tracking methods becomes vital in ensuring that you manage expectations while progressing safely. Engaging with fitness professionals can significantly support this. These experts possess a wealth of knowledge and experience in assessing individual capabilities and formulating tailored plans that work best for personal goals. For instance, a certified personal trainer can evaluate your current physical condition through assessments like body composition analysis or functional movement screenings. This process helps set a realistic foundation for what you can achieve, preventing overexertion and potential injuries.

It's not only about getting a coach to set your pace, it's about moral support and accountability. A lot of professionals will emphasize setting SMART (Specific, Measurable, Achievable, Relevant, Time-bound) goals, which is essential for building sustainable habits. They provide insight into your strengths or weaknesses or areas that might need cultivation into actionable goals. Let's say your goal is to run a 5K; a coach can outline actionable milestones to build towards that goal, such as adding a minute to your run-time every week or even integrating certain stamina-building exercises into your routine. In doing so, they make sure that these goals fit within your health conditions and fitness levels and provide that structure moving forward.

Regular consultations with these experts are key to adapting your approach as needed. Health and fitness are dynamic entities requiring periodic evaluation to stay on track. Checking in with a nutritionist might reveal if your diet supports your exercise regime or if modifications are necessary. A routine doctor's visit could highlight any new or persisting health concerns affecting your progress. Regularly seeking professional input can provide peace of mind knowing that safety is prioritized at every step. Furthermore, keeping communication open with fitness coaches allows adjustments to be made in response to life changes or unforeseen obstacles.

Once you've established initial guidelines through professional assistance, systematic monitoring of your workout routines and physical responses becomes essential. Keeping an exercise journal or using fitness apps can help track workouts, including details such as duration, intensity, and how you felt during and after. This information is invaluable when tweaking your exercise schedule, ensuring continuous growth without strain or injury. Analyzing trends over weeks or months can reveal patterns: Are there days when energy levels peak? Which exercises yield the most satisfaction and results? Knowing these answers aids in crafting a regimen that remains both effective and enjoyable.

Monitoring progress isn't just about tracking physical changes; it's also about staying in tune with your mindset. Sometimes, mental blocks or waning motivation can overshadow fitness achievements. This is where reconnecting with your "why" can be helpful. Remembering the reason you started your journey—whether it is improving your health, gaining confidence, or setting an example for loved ones—can help you push through challenges. Reflecting on your workouts and how they align with your purpose, perhaps through journaling, can also provide valuable insights into your emotional state and keep you motivated to stay on track.

For many, building a robust support system around these endeavors can be incredibly nurturing. Sharing experiences with peers creates a sense of camaraderie that bolsters commitment to self-improvement journeys. This network may consist of fellow gym-goers, friends participating in group classes, or even virtual communities dedicated to similar goals. Leveraging shared experiences leads to collective encouragement, making seemingly insurmountable tasks feel attainable and less intimidating.

Technology can certainly make tracking workout activity easier. Wearables such as fitness trackers or smartwatches continuously log data on heart rate, activity levels and sleep cycles. These tools deliver real-time feedback and help determine whether you're hitting your daily goals or should dial back on intensity. Going a step further, technology can help take the guesswork out of goal setting and can even introduce a social aspect that inspires people through what their peers are doing. This can build a competitive aspect of the fitness journey making workouts more fun.

One of the most important things to consider with any fitness program is the need for rest and recovery. It's repeated by professionals all the time that you need to listen to your body and not feel pressured to push yourself to the limit, every single day. Recovery does not have to be just resting muscles, it can includes things like stretching or yoga to release tension and improve flexibility. Complementing an active recovery with hydration, nutrition, and sleep optimizes performance while mitigating burnout risk. Along the way, milestones reached represent victories over obstacles — and a reaffirmation that even those with challenging histories can create lasting change.

Identifying Psychological Barriers

Stepping into a new fitness routine can be a daunting experience. Psychological barriers such as fear, anxiety, and self-doubt can significantly hinder progress toward fitness goals. Each step we take carries the risk of failure or the possibility of injury. Anxiety often stems from concerns about others' perceptions, which can lead individuals to withdraw from group activities. Similarly, self-doubt—a common feeling among those who have faced setbacks in the past—can undermine confidence and lead to giving up too easily.

In order to deal with these challenges, cognitive-behavioral techniques can be a practical choice. This consists of recognizing negative thought processes and turning them into positive affirmations. Instead of "I can't do this," you might think "I can tolerate discomfort." The change of mind set is tantamount to removing mental blocks and making the strongest of resilience. By actively practicing this technique over and over again, people can learn to deal with their fears and anxieties and clear the way for gradual progression.

Creating a support system is another effective way to combat these challenges. It creates a sense of belonging and removes the feeling of loneliness by connecting with people with similar goals. Such a network can consist of friends, family, or even online groups where people motivate one another and exchange experiences. Social support from communities around those passions is an important motivator and provides encouragement, accountability, and even a translation that says, hey, this matters! When people know they are supported and that they have people cheering them on, they're more likely to follow through with their plans and celebrate small wins on the way to their goal.

Shared experiences in these networks also normalize challenges, and help people feel less isolated in their struggles. Listening to stories of other people who have overcome those same walls is very powerful. It serves to reinforce the notion that setbacks are part of the process and not the end of it. Additionally, working with an accountability partner or group can elevate commitment levels; regular check-ins motivate individuals to follow through and remain focused on their goals.

Starting sobriety is a significant life change that involves both physical and mental adjustments. It's important to recognize the challenges that come with this transition, such as learning to handle stress without turning to substances. Fitness can be an excellent outlet for managing these pressures, as long as it's approached thoughtfully and with an understanding of your unique needs during this journey.

Gradual integration gives the mind and body time to adapt. Having realistic expectations and celebrating small successes help build self-esteem and fight against the self-blame. Simple habits such as journaling about situations, emotions and fitness-related thoughts can uncover trigger points or recurring patterns that need tackled. By openly acknowledging these moments (and without judgment) we develop a growth mindset and begin to cut through limiting beliefs.

Furthermore, it may be beneficial to consider professional support, such as counselling or therapy for anything fitness-related that is bothering you. Cognitive-behavioral therapy trained professionals can address how mental barriers can be counterproductive with individualized strategies to deal with stagnation mentally, so one can better manage stress and sustain motivation. For the hesitant starters or the uneasy continuers, knowing there's expert help to be had adds further reassurance to your day.

Mindfulness exercises can be found as complementary to fitness regimen that you can do together as well. Meditation, deep breathing and other practices lower anxiety levels, which help us feel calm enough to exercise. Such exercises improve focus and concentration and allow individuals to focus during workouts without being distracted by external pressure or internal doubts.

Regular engagement with these practices bridges the gap between mental intention and physical action, fostering a holistic well-being approach. Over time, participants will notice improved mood, increased energy, and greater clarity, which naturally encourages continued participation in fitness activities. The key is to make incremental and consistent steps instead of drastic sweeping changes.

The path to improved physical and mental health should be viewed as a marathon, not a sprint. It will take patience and perseverance though, change does not happen overnight. In this context, how are we framing the journey: positively, by focusing on the joys of progress, as opposed to the challenges along the way? A positive framing, aligns motivation with long-term vision. Centering on self-compassion helps put disappointments in perspective — reminding people that shortcomings are momentary and can be overcome..

Finally, embedding gratitude within this journey enhances overall satisfaction and resilience. Taking moments to reflect on one's efforts, acknowledging the strides made irrespective of magnitude, nurtures a positive relationship with fitness and self-improvement. Celebrating every milestone in our fitness journey and our sobriety instills pride and propels forward momentum.

Final Insights on Setting a Baseline

Understanding and evaluating both physical and mental health statuses are cornerstones for anyone embarking on a fitness journey, especially those navigating newfound sobriety or aiming to enhance overall well-being. This chapter has delved into the importance of recognizing unique physical constraints, emphasizing how personal factors such as past injuries or health conditions influence individual responses to exercise. The discussion highlighted the necessity of tailoring fitness routines that respect these limitations, promoting gradual progression while consulting professionals for personalized guidance. By acknowledging these needs, it's possible to create workout strategies that align with one's capabilities, ensuring safety and motivating positive outcomes.

Additionally, the mental landscape is equally pivotal in sustaining a successful fitness regimen. Identifying psychological barriers like fear, anxiety, and self-doubt, and addressing them through supportive communities or cognitive-behavioral techniques can foster resilience and motivation. This balanced approach ensures that both body and mind are prepared for change, leveraging mindfulness and community encouragement to transform challenges into stepping stones. By integrating monitoring practices and professional insights, individuals can continuously adapt and progress toward better health.

CHAPTER 6

Crafting a Personal Fitness Plan

In sobriety I have had the opportunity to do many things I would not have otherwise been able to do. One of the most impactful things was reclaiming my health. That has allowed me to do more things than I can count and every time I look in the mirror I am reminded of it. One of my most absolute favorite experiences ever was running the Disney Marathon. The excitement of running a big race is just indescribable and Disney knows how to put on a great show! There were fireworks, Disney characters, and crowds of people cheering us the whole way as we ran through each of the parks at Disney World. Along with not being drunk, having a training plan tailored to my goals is what made it possible.

My goal for the Disney Marathon was just to finish the entire race, because 26.2 miles is a long way. I did not care about time as much as I did about just being able to cross that finish line. To prepare for the marathon, I followed a training plan that I adapted to my own fitness level. It wasn't rocket science. I simply followed the recommendations of what others have done. Just like in getting sober, I followed the suggestions of those who had done it before me. What a novel idea!

A curious thing happened along the way in my marathon training that I did not expect. Because I knew where I was starting from physically and the plan was adapted to my needs, I became increasingly more and more driven to meet my milestones. In the past when I had overly ambitious ideas or vague plans without consideration for where I was starting from, I was unable to stay motivated because I was failing every target I set for myself. However, I had the exact opposite experience training for Disney. Because I could see the progress I was making against the plan I set in motion, I was able to stay committed to it. The plan was specific and realistic for what I was trying to do.

In this chapter, we cover the fundamentals of creating a tailored fitness plan designed for those in recovery from alcoholism in mind and to support overall well-being. Using tried-and-true techniques like the SMART criteria, you'll learn about structuring a fitness plan and set goals that are both achievable and inspiring. We will go step by step through creating short- and long-term goals that are flexible enough to accommodate the turns that life can throw at us but structured enough to give shape to the things that you accomplish. We will also cover how a supportive circle helps you stay on track and why you should celebrate all the achievements, big and small.

Setting Realistic Fitness Goals

One of the most important steps toward our health and wellness journey is developing a personal fitness plan that meets our own abilities and needs, and this is especially true for people new in recovery. So, it is very important to start with an honest assessment of the current fitness levels. This act is important in order to prevent you from having unrealistic expectations that could cause your frustration to lead to burnout. Knowing where you are physically will help you create goals that are attainable but not too easy, they should still push you to make progress. So, a fitness professional can be useful to help outline, assess the strengths and improvements. Furthermore, we can learn from past successes or past struggles.

Once you've gauged your baseline fitness, it's time to define your objectives using the SMART criteria: Specific, Measurable, Achievable, Relevant, and Time-bound. This structured approach ensures clarity and makes tracking your goals much easier. Specificity means honing in on precise targets, like running a particular distance or lifting a certain weight. Measurability allows you to track improvements, giving you tangible data to celebrate or learn from. Feasibility is about setting goals that stretch your capabilities without breaking them, ensuring sustainability. Relevance ties your aims to personal life circumstances and broader goals, thus increasing motivation. Lastly, establishing a timeline creates urgency and frames your journey within a manageable schedule. By adopting these guidelines, you set yourself up for success, creating clear pathways to your aspirations.

It's also vital to adapt your goals flexibly, allowing room for life's unpredictable nature. Progress isn't always linear; some days might be more challenging than others due to factors like stress or fatigue. Being too rigid can lead to discouragement when things don't go as planned. Instead, celebrate milestones and periodically reassess your objectives. For instance, if you're recovering from an injury or facing a busy time at work, modify workouts rather than abandoning them. This flexibility not only keeps you engaged but also builds resilience, helping maintain motivation during challenges.

Any well-balanced plan should have both short-term and long-term goals. Short-term goals serve as stepping stones, offering frequent opportunities for accomplishment. These might include weekly workout targets or monthly skill improvements, which keep motivation levels high by providing regular feedback. On the other hand, long-term goals are about envisioning the bigger picture—whether it's achieving a specific level of fitness or integrating exercise as a permanent part of your routine. These ambitions guide your overall direction and provide a sense of purpose. Setting both types of goals can create a dynamic plan that adapts and grows with you.

Building a support system around your fitness journey can also enhance commitment to your objectives. Engaging with friends, family, or a fitness community provides accountability and encouragement. Sharing goals with others can make them feel more real and less daunting, while the camaraderie offers emotional support during highs and lows. Additionally, consider pairing up with a workout buddy or joining group classes—these social elements not only add fun but also introduce external motivation. Making a commitment to meet someone at the gym will go along way toward keeping you on track when motivation is low.

Making progress gets you closer to your goal so it is important to recognize and appreciate your accomplishments, big and small. Every achievement reflects your hard work and dedication. Take stock of everything you've accomplished — big and small — and celebrate it. Whether it's treating yourself to some new piece of workout gear after hitting a milestone or simply milling over your hard work, these moments of celebration inspire continued engagement. They serve as a reminder of how far you've come and why you embarked on this path in the first place.

Incorporating Meaningful Milestones

Adding personally relevant targets to your fitness plan is a great way to increase commitment and stay on track. You will naturally hit unique milestones, and so aligning your exercise regime with these milestones can add serious motivation and commitment to the journey of recovery. Milestones should be something that hits close to home. These can range from doing a set amount of reps without stopping or hitting a certain personal best during a workout. When you focus your efforts on goals that have intrinsic value, you make it about more than just getting into physical shape — you make it about being a character in your own story, where you have ownership of the plot.

Every journey to recovery has its own story, and different experiences, feelings, and hopes along the way. Knowing what is important within this context taps into intrinsic motivation to make them a meaningful accomplishment rather than just a task. For some, personal milestones might be getting back some of the fitness lost to inactivity;

for others, it might be having the energy to hike with family again. Every milestone was a testimony of your journey, which motivated you to keep shoving those challenges that, one day, will help you accomplish the big goals.

Celebration is a key component in building positive momentum. Celebrating milestones along the journey is also a great motivator and builds engagement. Celebrations need not be extravagant; they can be genuine moments that validate your strength and your evolution. That might mean spending a day doing something you love, free from guilt, or telling a kind friend or mentor who recognizes your hard work about your success. The important thing is to stop and see how far you have come, no matter how small the progress is, because every step in the right direction is an achievement to be celebrated.

Celebrating wins gives you something concrete to point towards in terms of how far you have come and is a rewarding motivation to keep moving towards your end goals. The awareness creates good energy and a feedback mechanism where feeling accomplished after reaching the milestone encourages more accomplishments. It changes the process from a checklist of tasks into an experience of reminding yourself that you can change. Just as sobriety chips symbolize the milestones achieved (months and years) on the journey to recovery—each demonstrating perseverance and transformation—fitness milestones serve as markers of progress and commitment. Both represent tangible evidence of how far you've come—proof that small and consistent steps can lead to big changes.

Throughout this process, visualizing progress becomes a helpful tool as well, enabling you to see the tangible results of your hard work and dedication. A clear visualization of milestones reached and those still in progress can provide valuable insight into your journey. This might involve keeping a journal of daily reflections, using photos to document physical changes over time, or even plotting milestones on a calendar as visible reminders of your accomplishments. Having concrete evidence of your achievements will bolster confidence and inspire continued effort, particularly during challenging times.

While the focus remains on personal significance, avoid overwhelming yourself with complex guidelines. Instead, trust that understanding and recognizing the importance of integrating these personal milestones into your fitness plan will naturally enhance your commitment. Allow this process to unfold organically, respecting your unique rhythm and capacity for growth. Let each achievement serve as a beacon, guiding you closer to your recovery goals and reinforcing the ongoing narrative of your remarkable journey.

Visualizing Progress

Fostering accountability and inspiration in your personal fitness plan begins with effective tracking methods. Setting a goal without being able to measure progress is self-defeating from the start. It's like embarking on a journey without a map. This is where visual tools such as charts or journals come in handy. These tools are not just fancy gadgets; they serve a practical purpose, helping you keep a clear view of your progress towards your goals. By regularly updating your chart or journal, you stay connected with your objectives, continuously reminding yourself why you started this journey.

Visual aids play a key role in maintaining motivation, especially during challenging periods when enthusiasm may wane. They provide tangible proof of achievements that can bolster your morale. For example, seeing a graph line steadily rising or a journal filled with entries about completed workouts gives you undeniable evidence of your efforts and progress. This evidence can be very uplifting, serving as a reminder of how far you've come and reinforcing the belief that you can continue moving forward.

Moreover, regular tracking enables you to identify patterns in your exercise routine and results. Perhaps you notice that your energy levels dip at a certain time each day, or maybe you track more successful workouts when they occur in the morning versus the evening. Recognizing these patterns helps you make informed adjustments to enhance your results. It allows you to optimize your schedule for peak performance, ensuring that your exercise plan remains effective and aligned with your body's natural rhythms.

For those recovering from addiction or striving to improve their overall health, these tracking methods are particularly beneficial. As someone newly sober, integrating routine and structure into daily life can offer tremendous stability. Regular tracking and seeing consistent progress can help reinforce positive habits, providing a sense of control and accomplishment. Having clear evidence of success can also help combat feelings of self-doubt that might arise during recovery.

Imagine you're using a journal to track your workouts. Each entry could include details about the type of exercise, duration, intensity, and how you felt before and after the session. Over time, this journal becomes a rich source of information, reflecting your journey and milestones. You may discover that certain activities which seemed daunting at first gradually became easier, showcasing your physical improvements and resilience.

Charts, on the other hand, offer a different form of visualization. A simple graph tracking the number of minutes you exercise each week, increasing gradually, becomes a powerful visual testament to dedication and persistence. These charts are not static; they evolve alongside your fitness and recovery journey, continually adapting to highlight new accomplishments.

It's important to ensure that these tracking methods reflect not only your successes but also your learning experiences. Setbacks may happen, but they are opportunities to examine ourselves. When you encounter a period where progress stalls or seems to regress, use it as a chance to reassess and recalibrate your approach. Ask yourself what changes can be made to reignite momentum. Perhaps it's trying a new type of exercise, altering your schedule, or seeking additional support. The key is adaptability—a willingness to adjust and find what works best for you.

A second important aspect of effective tracking is accountability. Tracking your progress and sharing it with another trusted friend, family member or fitness group can help keep you accountable to your plan. Creating a support network around yourself just by the fact that people know of your goals and achievements. You get encouragement and constructive feedback on the track that keep you motivate more to stay on track.

Besides accountability, sharing your progress can inspire those who are starting similar journeys themselves. Your story — your challenges and triumphs in sobriety and fitness can be a ray of hope and motivation for others. No matter where you are in your journey, there is something you can offer as inspiration to others. Sharing your journey with others can not only be helpful to others but it can also serve as an additional tool to keep you motivated.

Final Insights on Personal Fitness Plans

Having a personalized fitness plan for yourself is vital, especially for those who may be aiming to improve their health from a long period of low activity or someone early sobriety. This chapter highlighted the importance of evaluating your fitness levels honestly, setting realistic goals using the SMART method, and maintaining flexibility in your objectives. By consulting with fitness professionals and reflecting on past experiences, you can design a plan that suits your unique capabilities while ensuring sustainability.

Moreover, integrating meaningful milestones into your routine enhances motivation and commitment. By aligning these milestones with personal recovery goals, you create a sense of ownership over your journey and transform exercise from a mere task into something significant. Acknowledging completed milestones, however small, creates an upward spiral, re-affirming the belief that you can do this. Visual tools to chart your progress like journals can also motivate you to continue when you see the amount of work you have put in. Having those things shared with a support system helps you internally visualize things and pushes you to do better, in so much as it helps those around improve as well on similar paths. Recognize that this process is only an additional step in your ongoing journey to be healthier and happier.

CHAPTER 7

Exercise and Emotional Well-being

Probably one of the most important skills that I learned in recovery, is how to better deal with the curveballs that life throws at us. Through the Twelve Steps, I learned how to better deal with stress and emotions. Particularly, I learned that whenever I look to something external to address uncomfortable feelings, I will always end up disappointed. I was sometimes able to find momentary comfort in food and alcohol but their effects were fleeting and the price I paid was far too high. In recovery, I found a toolkit for navigating life. As with any toolkit, different tools are appropriate for different tasks. Alcohol used to be my 'go to' method of making myself feel more relaxed, but in time it took more and more of it to achieve the same effect. At the same time the effects were diminishing, the consequences began to stack up. I would chase the calming effects I used to achieve with alcohol but would never find them again.

It was my Alcoholics Anonymous sponsor who introduced me to hot yoga. I was early in recovery and would often talk about the stress of my job and life. He suggested I try hot yoga. I would always have an excuse that I was too busy. I would comment that I used to be in really good shape and wanted to get back to that. He would suggest I try hot yoga. I didn't see how sitting around on the floor breathing and stretching would do anything for me other than waste time that I didn't have. Besides that, I wanted to get back in shape—so I told myself that I needed more than stretching.

I'm not sure if his suggestions just eventually wore me down or if it was simply curiosity, but I eventually went to a hot yoga class with my sponsor. I fell in love with it from the very first class. The room was 100 degrees with high humidity and I was asked to move into shapes that I didn't even know my body was capable of getting into. At the end of it, I think I had sweated a river out on the floor but the stress tension I had in my body when I left work was gone. I had a cold shower to cool down and felt positively euphoric. I had all of the same life issues that I had just 2 hours before, but I no longer felt any anxiety about it. Almost as if by magic, I just wasn't worried about any of it anymore. That night I slept like a baby.

Before I tried yoga, I thought I knew what it was all about. Like many, I had a preconceived notion that it was little more than a series of stretches, primarily practiced by those already flexible or seeking a serene, meditative experience. Much like the stereotypes I once held about alcoholism, my understanding of yoga was narrow and superficial. After coming to terms with the fact that I had an alcohol problem, I realized that alcoholics come in all shapes and sizes from all walks of life.

When I finally gave yoga a try, I realized it was much more than I had imagined. What surprised me most was its scalability. Yoga can meet you wherever you are in your fitness journey. It can be as gentle as a chair yoga session, suitable for someone recovering from an injury or someone elderly, or it can push the limits of strength and endurance in a way that challenges even professional athletes. I discovered that yoga is a discipline that strengthens the body, focuses the mind, and nurtures the spirit. It requires intention, balance, and the ability to be in the present—all things I struggled with in the chaos of my alcoholism.

Meditation on the other hand was something I understood a little better—even if at first, I was completely incapable of doing it. My first attempts were humbling. Quieting my mind felt impossible. I was used to constant chatter in my head with endless cycles of regret and anxieties. I would also constantly replay events of the day in my head. At first, sitting still with my thoughts was really very uncomfortable but I soon realized that discomfort was part of the process. Meditation wasn't about erasing thoughts but learning to observe them without judgment and let them pass. What truly amazed me was how yoga and meditation became invaluable tools in my sobriety toolkit.

Both yoga and meditation are powerful tools, which can play a key role in our recovery and fitness journeys, encouraging a deeper mind-body connection. Through these practices, people find different routes to healing that fall outside of conventional modes. The soft yet firm approach of yoga guides practitioners to a sense of steadiness and strength, while meditation provides a space for introspection and emotional regulation.

One of the best methods that help improve emotional well-being is the practice of doing exercises. Exercise, in addition to its physical benefits, has several important mental health benefits that are vital for anyone interested in managing stress effectively. Regular movement, woven into the fabric of daily life, is crucial for building core stability that lays the groundwork for the emotional resilience required to recover from trauma and support well-being. By exercising, individuals are able to harness tis powerful ability of endorphin release, mood enhancement, and diminished anxiety, which plays a huge role in the quest for a healthier mind.

This chapter explores various forms of exercises geared toward enhancing mood. It states that aerobic exercise — think running and cycling — is famous for its ability to lift your spirits because it boosts endorphin production. The psychological benefits of strength training, including enhanced self-esteem and confidence, are emphasized as are the group benefits of working out together in fitness classes, which provide social interaction and emotional support. Movements in the form of Tai Chi or yoga workouts provide whole body benefits by combining physical exertion with relaxation of the mind. Touching on the audible option accessible to the broader range of human fitness, this piece is intended as a holistic approach to integrate emotional growth & fortitude into the human experience that is your daily life.

Types of Exercises Beneficial for Mood Enhancement

Various types of workouts have their own unique properties that specifically improve mood and can even positively affect mental health. Now let's take a closer look at how these activities can change your mental state.

Aerobic exercises like running or cycling, which have been famous for raising endorphins, the body's natural feel good chemicals, are one way to begin. Endorphins are sometimes called "feel good" hormones because they can produce feelings of euphoria and happiness. Participating in regular aerobic exercise will boost your mood and decrease feelings of anxiety. People who integrate aerobic workouts into their weekly routines often say they feel more energized and less stressed. Not only do they instill a positive mindset, but they also help in building emotional resilience for the long term.

Another type of physical activity with profound psychological benefits is strength training. In addition to building muscle and improving physical strength, weightlifting or resistance training can significantly improve your body image, and your self-esteem. The confidence gained in seeing physical results can carry over to other areas of life with improved mental toughness and focus. For someone who is emerging from some previous struggles, developing physical strength becomes a metaphorical reminder that you have an incredible ability for dominance over adversity.

Group fitness classes are another way to boost your mood through community. In a world where isolation can seem palpable, particularly during recovery, group classes offer not only a venue for enhancing physical health, but also for creating bonds with others. Finding others on a similar fitness journey fosters connections that serve to remedy loneliness. Whether it's a yoga class, a spin session or a dance workout, the social element that's part of group activities can create a network of support, providing encouragement and friendship. The positive nature of these communal experiences builds emotional health, dissipating any remainders of separation.

Activities such as Tai Chi, yoga, and dance are mindful movements, where physical movements engage both mind and body, facilitating an easy and enjoyable whole body experience. Such practices highlight the connection between mind and body via gentle, flowing movement that demands focus and attention. They invite participants to breathe deeply, move slowly, letting go of stress, finding a meditative place. Mindful movement exercises help you be in the present, cleansing your mind of distractions, worries and anxieties. Regular practice may enhance emotional regulation, providing serenity and peace in a chaotic world.

Incorporating mindful exercises may also stimulate creativity and self-expression, and serve as a positive outlet for emotions. Moreover, these intensities are available to everyone, regardless of fitness, which makes them an ideal option for anyone who wants to be in a better state but does not want to go through wear and tear workouts. Whether you adhere to a workout program every day or find that you cannot muster up enough energy or time to do anything more than a walk around the block, find ways to make exercise a part of your everyday life — to incorporate it into your daily routine. Aerobic workouts, when viewed as achievements, serve as key moments of success in one's recovery journey, fortifying emotional resilience by demonstrating personal growth and overcoming hurdles effectively. Participants actively engaging in consistent aerobic exercises frequently notice heightened energy levels alongside diminished stress, empowering them to face various emotional challenges with a refreshed mindset.

To make this integration successful, start small, gradually building intensity and duration, and choose activities you genuinely enjoy. Mix and match different types of exercises to keep things interesting and to reap varied benefits. Celebrating small victories along the way reinforces commitment and motivation, making exercise a habitual and enjoyable component of daily life. Strength training sessions not only sculpt your physique but bolster your self-image, nurturing newfound mental fortitude that permeates through life's trials. Joining group fitness classes unlocks a treasure trove of camaraderie and support, knitting a safety net against isolation that simultaneously uplifts your spirits through mutual achievements.

Mindful movements, acting as soothing balms to frazzled nerves, systematically unwind stress while sharpening focus, bestowing peace and balance upon practitioners. Infuse exercise seamlessly into your lifestyle by consistently scheduling sessions that align with your needs. Combining technology's prowess, leveraging apps, and tapping into online communities conjure accountability and trail progress, freeing up motivation and enthusiasm as you traverse this transformative venture. Especially in recovery, exercise's role is more than just physiology. It stands as a cornerstone in the foundation of emotional and physical well-being.

Strategies for Consistent Practice

Exercise is one of the best tools to help manage stress and think clearly — both of which are invaluable for those new to sobriety, with many seeking ways to improve their mental health. Grounding yourself in this habit on a daily basis can serve as the discipline you seek for emotional regulation. In order to get into a consistent routine with working out, one of the best things you can do is to pick a specific time to work out. Having specific timeframes set aside for physical exercise eliminates procrastination and prevents immobility. As with any new pattern, the magic is in the regularity, so integrating movement as a non-negotiable aspect of day-to-day life elevates it from some task to cross off the to-do list into a cornerstone of the self-care process.

Imagine waking up every morning at the same time to go for a jog or heading to the gym after work as part of a ritual. These activities not only contribute to physical fitness but also instill a sense of accomplishment that resonates throughout the day. For those recovering from addiction, having such structured routines can replace old habits with healthier ones, providing a positive framework. Establishing a regular schedule also serves as a reliable anchor in times of emotional upheaval, offering predictability and familiarity, which are comforting amid life's uncertainties.

While setting a schedule lays the groundwork, discovering activities that captivate you personally can significantly boost motivation. Whether it's dancing, swimming, or cycling, engaging in exercises that resonate with you adds enjoyment to the routine. When a workout feels less like a chore and more like recreation then people are naturally more inclined to keep at it. This personal resonance can transform the way one views exercise—not so much as a necessity but rather as a cherished hobby. Therefore, exploring different physical activities to find what truly excites you can be a rewarding process. Participating in something enjoyable makes it easier to commit long-term, leading to sustained engagement and improved emotional health.

Once a form of exercise has been chosen and embraced, allowing for small peaks in performance can help maintain high levels of interest and motivation to train. These milestones serve as tangible markers of progress, offering a clear sense of direction on the fitness journey. They can range from gradually increasing running distances to mastering a new yoga pose. By defining incremental steps to success, these milestones enable more frequent celebrations of progress. Acknowledging small wins reinforces positive behaviors, as team members focus on their achievements. This not only boosts the overall morale of the group but also creates a motivating cycle that encourages continued participation. Engaging in this process fosters a sense of competence and confidence, equipping individuals to tackle other aspects of life with a renewed sense of purpose.

Along with creating milestones, tracking progress is extremely helpful. Tracking workouts, in a journal, app or calendar, is literal proof of progression over time. Not only does this provide accountability—seeing evidence of consistency can motivate people through difficult days—it in itself is a form of motivation. Taking a look back at how far someone has come during their fitness journey, serves as a strong reminder of what one is capable of accomplishing. When you wake up tired or feeling unworthy a record of your previous accomplishments can spark determination again.

Visual trackers or even digital apps offer practical means of monitoring advancement. They not only chart progress but can introduce an element of gamification, making exercise more engaging by setting challenges or awarding badges for consistency. The gratification of ticking off completed tasks or reaching a new level can be immensely satisfying and motivational. Moreover, tracking brings attention to areas needing improvement, allowing for adjustments in routines to optimize results.

Integrating Exercise into Daily Life

When juggling lots of other responsibilities it can seem overwhelming to add something new—such as an exercise routine. To make this transition smoother, begin with small time commitments. This approach helps build a habit without feeling like an additional burden. For instance, starting with just ten minutes of physical activity each day can be enough to lay the groundwork for a more prolonged fitness regimen. Over time, these short sessions can gradually extend as you become more comfortable and find your rhythm. Consistency is key here—regularity, even in small doses, can significantly impact emotional well-being by reducing stress levels and improving mood stability.

Incorporating technology can also play a vital role in maintaining consistency and motivation. Fitness apps offer numerous features that help track progress, set goals, and provide reminders. Many apps allow you to personalize workout plans based on available time and preferred activities. Furthermore, online communities associated with these apps create spaces where users can share achievements, seek advice, and offer encouragement. This sense of community provides accountability, motivating individuals to maintain their routines and celebrate milestones.

One effective way to enhance both the enjoyment and sustainability of exercising is through social engagement. Involving family members or friends in your workouts transforms fitness into a shared activity and experience. This approach not only adds an element of fun but also boosts motivation and strengthens relationships. Whether it's taking a daily walk with your partner or attending a weekly yoga class with a friend, exercising together can make the experience feel less like a chore and more like a social outing. Training alongside others who share similar goals fosters connections that can help keep you on track.

Allowing for flexibility in your schedule can help with sustainability. Life is unpredictable, and a rigid schedule may not always be attainable in daily life, making you feel frustrated or even discouraged. By tailoring exercises around your own personal lifestyle, you can make sure that the routine can be number feel like a challenge. This could also mean opting for workouts that you can do at home, so bodyweight workouts or using resistance bands means you can work out without needing access to certain equipment or a gym. Or for the time-strapped out there, making way to do exercise alongside something else — such as cycling to work or having walking meetings — can help you to weave physical activity into your day without too much disruption.

For many, a feeling of inclusion can also help with struggling with loneliness when going through tough times like a recovery. By joining groups, you not only feel part of the community but also triggers a sense of help among each other. Shared experiences in physical exercise can create deeper connections between those involved, offering you a network of peers who relate and understand what you are going through. The added benefits of motivation and encouragement are often found in group classes. Seeing others continue to push through can encourage you to succeed, fostering both physical fitness and emotional strength.

Final Thoughts on Exercise and Emotional Well-Being

We learned in this chapter about the importance of incorporating many types of exercise into your daily routine, for the sake of emotional health and stress management benefits. From endorphin-releasing workouts building emotional resilience to self-esteem-building strength training to community connection through groups—every approach offers unique contributions to emotional health. In addition, mindful motion such as Tai Chi releases stress and can bring about a profound state of calm and equilibrium. Doing these exercises regularly also helps rewire your environment for being constructive instead of destructive, contributing to recovery and growth by replacing bad habits with good ones.

Find something enjoyable and begin with small consistent steps. When you establish realistic goals, track your progress, and celebrate significant milestones along the way, you will feel more focused and dedicated. Whether you prefer to get out there for a run or sign up for a group class, make working out a treasured part of your daily routine, providing you with both the physical benefits and emotional stability needed in this uncertain time. Combining both consistency with enjoyment, this will help to make exercise less of a task and more of a vehicle to improving mental health and helping you get through life.

CHAPTER 8

Nutrition 101 – Back to Basics

Sadly, I was over 30 years old before I realized that the old cliché about "you are what you eat" was more than a catchy phrase—it is a biological fact. Literally every cell in your body is constructed from the raw materials you consume. Your muscles, bones, skin, and organs are all formed and maintained by the nutrients supplied through your diet. If your diet consists of nutrient-rich, high-quality foods, your body has the building blocks it needs to thrive. But if your meals are dominated by potato chips, cheese puffs, and sugary sodas, your body is left trying to build itself out of fluff. It's a bit like attempting to construct a skyscraper from cotton candy and marshmallows—maybe appropriate for a carnival, but disastrous for structural integrity.

Imagine the intricate systems of your body as a construction site. Your muscles need protein to repair and grow, much like steel beams are necessary to support a building. Your bones require calcium and vitamin D to stay strong, akin to the concrete foundation of a skyscraper. Healthy skin, organs, and connective tissue rely on vitamins, minerals, and healthy fats, just as a building depends on high-quality wiring and insulation. Without these essential components, the body cannot operate efficiently or achieve its full potential.

A diet of processed, sugary foods might provide temporary energy and satisfaction, but it doesn't deliver the raw materials needed for strength, endurance, or resilience. Over time, this leads to fatigue, poor performance, and a body that struggles to maintain itself. On the other hand, a diet rich in lean proteins, whole grains, vegetables, and healthy fats equips your body with the resources it needs to thrive. A body that is healthy and thriving is simply more capable of dealing with the transition from active alcoholism to a life without it. This just makes sense much the same way that the building blocks of what makes up our body comes from what we eat.

In addition to being the building blocks of everything our body is made of, our diets are also the fuel for everything we do. It provides the energy needed to power everything. This is especially important when adjusting to a new life beyond alcohol in which we aspire to a more physically active lifestyle. If we attempt to have a physically active lifestyle, then we need the fuel to do it. Without that fuel our intensity will be diminished in our workouts and we simply will not achieve optimal results. Our everyday routines will also be negatively impacted. Imagine a flashlight with a battery nearly dead compared to one with a new and fully charged battery.

In active alcoholism and addiction we often placed more emphasis on feeding our addiction than we did to feeding our bodies of the nutrients it needed to function properly. As a result, we found ourselves depleted of essential elements. Overcoming addiction is a process that involves much more than willpower—it also requires nourishing the body with proper nutrition to restore and reinvigorate it. But this chapter starts with the understanding that nutrition goes far beyond counting calories or hopping on the latest dietary fad; it is about making choices that will facilitate long-term health and by extension recovery.

In this chapter, we will cover planning out our meals to support sustained energy and keep our mood stable. We hope to arm you with the tools you need to make informed dietary choices that will help you on your pathway to sobriety. A diet that gives your body the support it needs to heal isn't complicated or rigid—it's about you having the knowledge to make simple, meaningful swaps to nourish your healing body and putting that plan into action.

Key Nutrients to Support Healing

Nutrition plays a pivotal role in achieving and maintaining health. Proper nutrition provides the body with the essential nutrients needed to repair, rebuild, and sustain itself, creating a foundation for physical and mental well-being. Good health, supported by a balanced diet, enhances the body's ability to recover, improves energy levels, stabilizes mood, and fosters resilience—critical elements in the journey of recovery. By prioritizing nutrition, you are equipping yourself with a vital tool to strengthen your progress and support lasting sobriety.

Among the key dietary elements that play an important role in our bodies is protein. Proteins serve as the building blocks of life, supporting the structure, function, and repair of cells and tissues throughout the body. Incorporating adequate, high-quality protein into your diet can promote overall health by aiding in muscle maintenance, supporting immune function, and contributing to better mental clarity. By ensuring a balanced intake of protein along with other nutrients, you can help create a foundation for improved energy levels, mood stability, and a greater sense of well-being.

To meet your protein needs, recommended dietary sources include lean meats, fish, eggs, dairy products, beans, nuts and seeds. Aside from playing roles in tissue repair, these sources play key roles in neurotransmitter functions that affect mood. Lean meats, such as chicken and turkey, are high in amino acids (the precursors to serotonin and dopamine, which affect mood and cognition). Fish, especially fatty types, such as salmon, offer omega-3 fatty acids along with protein so you get brain- and inflammation-fighting benefits all in one. Introducing these elements to one's plate can pave the way for good mental health habits.

In tandem with macronutrients, protein, vitamins and minerals also provide a foundation of nutrition recovery here. Different vitamins like B-complex and vitamin C and minerals like magnesium and zinc can work wonders for health in general including brain function. At this point, you may have already guessed that these nutrients are critical in relation to stress reduction, mood, and cognitive function. Vitamin B-complex vitamins (B1 or thiamine, B6 or pyridoxine, and B12 or cobalamin) are especially crucial as they contribute to the maintenance of a healthy nervous system. Moreover, alcoholism frequently results in shortages of these vitamins with which it must be replenished. Whole grains, legumes, leafy green vegetables and fortified cereals can provide these essential vitamins.

Vitamin C has immune boosting properties and plays multiple roles in our health. It has antioxidant properties and helps combat oxidative stress which can be induced by alcohol consumption. Citrus fruits, strawberries, bell peppers and broccoli are just some sources of vitamin C and are easily incorporated into daily diets. Minerals like magnesium and zinc are just as critical, though. Magnesium helps for the transmission of nerves and the relaxation of muscles, which helps you reduce anxiety and sleep better, while zinc provides immune support and promotes wound healing. These minerals are rich in nuts, seeds, whole grains, all strongly associated with general well-being and mental acuity.

The role of healthy fats should not be discounted as they play a pivotal role in reducing inflammation, supporting mental health, increasing satiety, balancing hormones and helping with nutrient absorption. One group of particularly promising nutrients are omega-3 fatty acids (which are abundant in fish oils, walnuts, chia seeds, and flaxseeds) that have been reported to have a significant impact on brain health. These fats help mitigate inflammatory processes inside the brain that can be aggravated by alcohol abuse. Inclusion of these sources in the diet can enhance mood and cognitive flexibility, as crucial in learning to deal with recovery.

In addition, fats promote the absorption of fat-soluble vitamins — A, D, E, and K — that are essential for dozens of processes in the human body, such as vision, bone health, antioxidant protection, and blood clotting. Including wholesome fats into a meal can therefore promote the wholesome efficient absorption of nutrients. These beneficial fats can also contribute to hormonal balance, which can further help stabilize mood swings when we're in recovery, so adding avocado, olive oil, and oily fish into meals helps to achieve this.

One of the most overlooked components of overall nutrition is adequate hydration. Water is essential for nearly every function in the body, from supporting detoxification processes and regulating body temperature to improving cognitive function and stabilizing mood. Proper hydration also plays a key role in maintaining healthy skin, aiding digestion, and ensuring optimal physical performance. The amount of water each person needs can vary based on factors like activity level, time of day, and environmental conditions, but aiming for around eight to ten glasses a day is a good general guideline. Making hydration a priority helps keep your body functioning at its best, contributing to overall vitality and well-being.

Meal Planning for Balanced Nutrition

Knowing the macronutrient breakdown of your meals is at the heart of building a balanced plate, which is key to keeping your energy and mood on an even keel. Staying active during recovery can be very helpful for overall mood and as we already know, food is the fuel for everything we do. Each macronutrient — carbohydrates, proteins, and fats — provides different benefits that together make up a balanced meal. Carbohydrates are your body's primary source of energy, proteins support tissue repair and muscular growth, while fats are necessary for absorbing vitamins and keeping cells healthy.

One approach for making balancing these nutrients easier is using a visual guide, such as the "plate method." Visual guides can help you portion your plate: half full of vegetables and fruits, a quarter with protein sources and a quarter with whole grains or starchy vegetables. This simple method helps you ensure you are getting the right proportions without having to measure everything out religiously.

Meal prep doesn't have to mean preparing an entire week's worth of meals in advance—it can be as simple as organizing basic ingredients for a few days and keeping them in one designated area of the kitchen. Having pre-planned, convenient options eliminates the stress of deciding what to eat, especially on busy days or when energy is running low. By taking a little time to prepare ahead, you can ensure that healthy, satisfying choices are always within reach. This approach not only saves time but also helps you stay consistent with your nutrition goals by making it easy to avoid less healthy, last-minute decisions.

Although, a tried-and-true way to go about meal prepping is to dedicate one day a week — maybe Sunday or whatever works for you — to cooking up a week's worth of meals. Alternatively, start by preparing simple recipes that use similar ingredients. Roast chicken, for example, can be repurposed into salads, wraps or even stir-fry. This both reduces waste and adds variety without a huge effort.

Dietary diversity is also crucial for preventing nutrient deficiency and keeping meals interesting. A variety of foods on your plate exposes you to a wider range of nutrients that are important for overall health and recovery. Experimenting with different cuisines or seasonal produce adds new flavors and keeps your diet from growing stale. Plus, the variety of vegetables, fruits, whole grains, and proteins means you are more likely to receive the key vitamins and minerals that you need to be operating at your peak.

It does not have to be intimidating to include variety. Start small, for example, trying one new fruit or vegetable each week. Or try some international recipes, which can sometimes teach you a new combination of foods, which can somewhat expand your taste buds and increase the nutritional value of your meal as well.

In addition to variety, mindful eating can be very helpful with how much we eat. When being mindful about food consumption it creates a much better relationship with food, encourages awareness of what we eat. Because you fully focus on the food you eat, you get to taste and enjoy every single bite, which naturally takes your digestion a level up.

Setting the table away from distractions such as TV or mobile devices promotes slower, more mindful eating, which makes us more aware of our hunger and fullness cues.

To practice mindful eating at mealtime, start with clearing away distractions and savor the sensory experience of food — its smell, texture, taste, even its visual appeal. Eat mindfully—chew your food slowly and taste every mouthful. Not only is this better for digestion but it improves your overall satiety and lowers the chance that you'll overeat or grab unhealthy snacks an hour after you're done eating.

Final Thoughts on Nutrition

In this chapter we looked at how a balanced diet plays a crucial role in supporting overall health and well-being. Nutrients like proteins, vitamins, minerals, and healthy fats are essential allies in maintaining both physical and mental resilience. Proteins help repair tissues and sustain energy levels, which are vital for endurance and focus. Vitamins and minerals support a vast array of functions in the body and enhance immune function. By prioritizing these nutrients, you empower your body to function optimally, paving the way for long-term health and vitality.

In addition, drinking plenty of fluids and eating a wide variety of whole foods can help support health and recovery. Healthy fats support brain function and mood regulation, and hydration helps your body process these nutrients efficiently and effectively. So as you incorporate these dietary changes, know that they work together not only for your immediate but also your long-term goals. This conceptualization of nourishment builds a stronger foundation for holistic healing with a recovery that restores the connection between mind and body.

CHAPTER 9

The Importance of Rest

Quality sleep is one of the most critical aspects of health, yet when I was drinking, it was also one of the most neglected. I often used my inability to sleep as an excuse to drink, convincing myself that alcohol would help me relax and drift off. But the reality was far from that. I didn't really fall asleep—I passed out. And passing out is not the same thing as restorative sleep. Passing out is the body shutting down, not recharging.

True sleep is a vital process that allows your body and mind to heal, reset, and prepare for the next day. When I was drinking, Despite the four hours or so of unconsciousness at night that I would get, I was in a constant state of sleep deprivation. Instead of waking up feeling rested, I often crawled out of bed feeling groggy, irritable, and even more exhausted. Toward the end of my drinking the shaking from withdraws had become so bad that I would need a shot of something to drink immediately upon waking just to be able to function. Looking back on it, I'm not sure how I managed to hide my problem from the world as long as I did.

In sobriety, I've learned that quality sleep is a cornerstone of health and wellness. This chapter explores the vital connection between sleep, fitness, and sobriety, offering insights into how to establish a healthier relationship with rest and why it's so critical for long-term health.

When we think about physical transformation from exercise, the focus often falls on daytime activities—hours spent in the gym, the intensity of our workouts, or the muscles we target. While these efforts are important, they're only part of the equation. The real transformation happens during sleep. This is when the body repairs itself: muscles rebuild, hormones balance, and energy stores are replenished. During strength training microscopic tears in muscle fibers occur, a necessary stress that triggers the body to rebuild stronger. Without sufficient rest, however, this recovery process is incomplete, leaving progress stalled and the body vulnerable to injury and fatigue.

Prolonged alcohol use compounds this challenge by disrupting neurotransmitter balance, which interferes with the body's natural sleep cycles. Alcohol's sedative effects may make it easier to fall unconscious, but it also suppresses REM sleep and disrupts the deeper stages of restorative sleep. Over time, this leaves the body and mind deprived of the essential time needed for revitalization. Alcohol also depresses the central nervous system. Prolonged use of alcohol will cause a rebounding effect once it is removed. This rebounding effect is responsible for many of the withdraw symptoms experienced when we first quit drinking. As a result, sleep in early recovery can be especially challenging. Thankfully, this effect is temporary and will subside once balance is restored in the central nervous system.

This chapter will delve into the multidimensional impact of sleep on fitness. You'll learn how quality sleep supports better decision-making, emotional stability, and stress management—key components in helping avoiding relapse and maintaining a sober lifestyle. We'll explore the consequences of poor sleep and the numerous benefits of restorative rest, from bolstering your immune system to regulating hormones. Along the way, you'll gain practical strategies to improve your sleep habits, empowering you to achieve your recovery and fitness goals with renewed strength and focus.

Impact of Sleep on Recovery Outcomes

Sleep deprivation can lead to a cascade of negative effects on emotional and mental well-being. When the body doesn't get enough rest, it disrupts the balance of hormones that influence mood, such as serotonin, dopamine, and cortisol. This imbalance can result in irritability, feelings of sadness, and heightened emotional reactivity. Additionally, the lack of restorative sleep puts the body in a state of stress, increasing levels of cortisol, the stress hormone. Over time, this can lead to persistent feelings of anxiety and overwhelm, making it harder to cope with daily challenges. The combination of low mood and elevated stress not only impacts mental clarity but can also affect relationships, motivation, and overall quality of life. High-quality sleep is essential for maintaining emotional balance and reducing the physical and mental toll of stress. As anyone in recovery from substance use can tell you, emotions can fluctuate wildly in early recovery. In such a state, quality sleep serves as a stabilizer to regulate our emotions.

One important area impacted by this is mental clarity. A good night's sleep enables the brain to process information more effectively, improving focus and allowing for calm, well-informed decision-making. This enhanced decision-making ability is especially important during recovery, where navigating complex situations with clarity and understanding is crucial. In recovery, it is often strongly suggested that we avoid making big life-changing decisions as much as practically possible during the first year after quitting drinking. This suggestion comes from practical lessons learned from those who have stopped drinking before us.

Sleep deprivation does not just make you feel tired and less resilient to stress but it also adds to your stress level. Stress creates a strain on the body's systems damaging both mental and physical health. Mental wellness is an essential component of recovery. Sleep supports mental health by providing the brain the downtime it needs to reset, processing emotions and experiences in a constructive manner. This mental reset is crucial in preventing the feeling of being overwhelmed, giving you the capacity to engage positively with your recovery process. Combining improved immune function and hormonal balance with enhanced mental wellness forms a comprehensive support system for anyone aiming for long-term sobriety.

There's a direct correlation between disrupted sleep patterns and substance use, a cycle that can self-perpetuate. Irregular sleep schedules often go hand-in-hand with the chaotic lifestyle associated with substance use. Breaking free from this cycle requires establishing consistent routines. Consistency in sleeping habits grounds your day-to-day life, setting a rhythm that supports healing and abstinence. A stable routine helps regulate your internal clock, and by aligning your sleep schedule with natural bodily rhythms, you increase your chances of successful recovery substantially. A structured routine imparts a sense of normalcy, gradually distancing you from past behaviors. Over time, this regularity strengthens your resolve, diminishes the chaos alcohol use introduced, and supports a healthier, balanced lifestyle conducive to long-term well-being.

Techniques to Improve Sleep Quality

Creating an ideal sleep environment is the first step towards improving sleep quality, which as we have already covered plays a significant role in recovery. This environment should be designed to facilitate the natural progression of sleep cycles. For most people, darkness signals the brain that it's time to rest. This means minimizing artificial light exposure from sources like phones, televisions, and computers close to bedtime. In our modern digital world, this is something many people struggle with.

Noise can also be a disruptive factor. Even subtle sounds can disturb the depth and continuity of sleep. Therefore, using earplugs or white noise machines can counteract these effects. Room temperature can also be an issue. The ideal temperature varies from person to person, but generally, cooler environments are recommended for optimal sleep. The key thing is being comfortable.

Establishing a consistent sleep routine is another important component of enhancing sleep quality. Our bodies thrive on regularity. Going to bed and waking up at the same time every day, even on weekends, can help reinforce our body's natural sleep-wake cycle. Setting this rhythm helps signal your body when it's time to rest and when to wake, optimizing your sleep quality. To successfully adhere to a routine, it can be beneficial to carve out a pre-sleep ritual. This can serve as a cue to your body and mind that it's time to wind down. Activities such as reading a book, taking a warm bath, or engaging in gentle stretching exercises can be relaxing. Avoiding stimulants like caffeine or nicotine, particularly in the hours leading up to bedtime, can also help in this process.

Mindfulness and relaxation techniques can be very helpful in preparing the mind for restful sleep. Often, anxiety and overthinking are barriers to falling asleep easily as we replay the events of the day in our heads or worry about other things that may happen tomorrow. Mindfulness practices such as meditation or deep-breathing exercises can help calm these thoughts. It will require practice, but by focusing on the present moment and letting go of these thoughts, mindfulness can reduce mental clutter and make it easier to drift into sleep. Guided meditations available through apps or audio recordings can be very helpful for those new to the practice, teaching users how to let go of the thoughts that do not serve us to relax and fall asleep.

Finally, monitoring sleep habits can offer valuable insights into what might be affecting your sleep quality. When all else fails, keeping a sleep journal or using a sleep-tracking app can help identify patterns and potential issues. Pay particular attention to the activities prior to sleep, any disruptions during the night, and your mood upon waking. Make sure to take note of when you last ate before bed and when you put down electronic devices. Over time, these records may reveal trends, such as how certain foods or how artificial light affects your sleep cycle.

This information can be crucial in adjusting habits or seeking professional guidance to address persistent sleep issues. If sleep disturbances continue despite these efforts, consulting a healthcare provider may uncover underlying conditions like sleep apnea or persistent insomnia, which may require some form of medical intervention.

Understanding Sleep Patterns and Their Role in Recovery

Each person's individual sleep needs and patterns vary, but in general the experts recommend a minimum of 6 to 8 hours daily. Recognizing your unique sleep needs can play a part in tailoring a recovery plan that aligns with your new lifestyle. This tailored approach not only supports physical rejuvenation but also enhances mental clarity. For instance, some individuals may find they need less sleep than the recommendations and still feel productive, while others require more hours to function optimally. Identifying these personal variations helps in creating an effective recovery strategy that minimizes the risk of relapse by promoting well-rested minds and bodies.

Disruptions in sleep have far-reaching effects beyond just feeling tired. A lack of quality sleep can affect both physical and mental health, which in turn impacts recovery strategies negatively. Sleep deprivation can exacerbate feelings of anxiety or depression, making it harder to focus on sobriety goals. Physically, it may lead to weakened immune responses or increased vulnerability to illness. This interplay between disrupted sleep and overall well-being means that addressing sleep issues should be a priority in any comprehensive recovery plan. Studies consistently show that proper sleep aids in reducing stress levels, improving mood, and enhancing cognitive functions, all of which are essential in sustaining recovery.

Establishing a consistent sleep routine is another critical component for those seeking long-term sobriety success. Having regular sleep and wake times helps in aligning the body's internal clock, known as the circadian rhythm. When this rhythm is disrupted, it can lead to various health problems. By going to bed and waking up at the same time every day, even on weekends, you reinforce your body's natural rhythms and promote better rest. Consistency becomes a foundation upon which other healthy habits can be built, providing structure and stability in everyday life that fosters long-term recovery.

Proper sleep hygiene is an important factor to understand. Sleep hygiene refers to the things we do that contribute to quality rest, such as maintaining a comfortable sleeping environment, avoiding caffeine before bed, and engaging in relaxing pre-sleep activities. These practices help in building resilience against stressors related to recovery. For example, lowering screen time before bed helps reduce exposure to blue light, which can hinder sleep quality. Understanding and implementing good sleep hygiene practices can minimize night-time waking and improve the continuity of sleep, ensuring that you wake up feeling refreshed and ready to face daily challenges.

Research shows that sleep interruptions can have an immediate impact on recovery results. For those in recovery from alcohol use disorder, disruptions in sleep can be a major hurdle given the need for the central nervous system to rebalance itself immediately after quitting drinking. The interplay of sleep and mood is complex, poor sleep can promote irritability and mood swings, states not supportive of recovery. Understanding these connections can help direct people to sleep-related interventions in adjunct to traditional treatment modalities.

As best you can, stick to a regular sleep schedule. A regular sleep routine will help regulate circadian rhythms and also offers a sense of normalcy. This sense of predictability and structure is often lacking in the early stages of recovery, making it all the more important to establish routines wherever possible. Sleep schedules provide a daily anchor, helping to regulate emotions and decrease impulsivity, which are common triggers for relapse. Slowly, as the routine becomes habit, individuals notice improved mood regulation and enhanced energy levels, both of which are crucial for navigating the complexities of life after alcohol.

Final Insights on Rest

In this chapter, we've explored how crucial adequate sleep is for re-covery and overall well-being. Sleep is not just a time for rest; it's an essential component that helps your body and mind recover, making it easier to handle life's challenges. Adequate sleep promotes cognitive clarity, enhances emotional stability and bolsters immune function. These benefits are critical for promoting stress management and pre-venting relapse to old habits. And by understanding and addressing sleep and related issues, we can promote a supportive environment for continued recovery and well-being. Adequate sleep enhances cognitive clarity, emotional regulation and immune function. These benefits are crucial for reducing stress and preventing people from returning to their former habits. When we recognize and manage sleep problems, we can lay the groundwork for long-term recovery and health.

Creating regular sleep routines and practicing healthy sleep hygiene can significantly enhance overall sleep quality. Establishing a consistent sleep schedule is crucial; small yet impactful steps, such as keeping con-sistent sleep-wake times and cultivating a soothing bedtime routine, can lead to substantial improvements in how well you sleep. These routines can include activities such as dimming the lights, engaging in relaxing activities like reading or gentle stretching, and minimizing screen time before bed.

in addition to these beneficial practices, being acutely aware of your individual needs and unique patterns of sleep can empower you to con-struct a comprehensive recovery plan that is specifically tailored to suit your lifestyle. Understanding whether you are a night owl or an early bird, for example, can influence your sleep strategy and help you opti-mize your rest.

Healthy sleep habits can be customized to align with an individual's lifestyle, encouraging choices that seamlessly integrate into both the re-covery process and daily life. This holistic approach not only aids in im-proving sleep but also fosters better overall well-being.

Ultimately, making sleep a priority in your life is an empowering step toward fostering a healthier and more balanced lifestyle, especially in our fast-paced world where the demands of work, family, and social obligations often take precedence. Prioritizing rest can ultimately lead to enhanced productivity, better emotional health, and a greater sense of vitality, allowing individuals to thrive in all aspects of their lives.

CHAPTER 10

Building a Supportive Environment

One of the suggestions in Alcoholics Anonymous is that we become part of a homegroup. A homegroup in Alcoholics Anonymous is the meeting a member chooses to call their "home" for their recovery journey. It's more than just a regular meeting; it's a place where members build deeper connections, contribute to the group's functioning, and receive consistent encouragement. Being part of a homegroup provides a sense of stability and accountability, as members often rely on each other for support, guidance, and sharing experiences.

One day early in sobriety, I was unable to make it to the meeting that I called my homegroup. That meeting was held once a week after work and several of us would also get together afterwards for food and fellowship. When I didn't show up for the meeting this particular night, the other homegroup members became concerned for me. I started getting multiple texts and phone calls telling me to get myself to the meeting. In the moment I was thoroughly annoyed, but I also became keenly aware that those guys genuinely cared about my welfare. If I had been in the beginning of a relapse, they were going to hunt me down and do whatever was within their power to stop me. I realized just how much I could count on them to help me stay sober. I was oddly annoyed and grateful at the same time. I will never forget the experience. I will also never again miss the meeting without letting everyone know that I can't make it.

This chapter emphasizes the power of connection and community in encouraging our lifestyle changes. By fostering an atmosphere where your health goals are understood and supported by family and friends, individuals can cultivate a network that enhances motivation and resilience. Supportive environments are not just beneficial—they're essential for sustaining long-term progress. Individuals often find that when they share their journey with others, the encouragement and empathy they receive become powerful motivators on days when personal resolve wavers.

Another focus of the chapter is practical ways to move supporters from passive to active roles, building active partnerships that serve to amplify both fitness and sobriety efforts. Readers will also find insight on how to get family and friends on board with our wellness plans, and how that can lead to a positive change in relationships in general. Readers will learn, from enjoying shared activities to establishing shared goals to celebrating milestones together, how a collaborative process can inject freshness and spice into the day-to-day experience. Through exploring the reciprocal advantages that a supportive network yields, this chapter allows readers to tap into the shared strength of their social circles.

Involving Family and Friends

Getting family and friends involved in your recovery can be an important part of the process. Being transparent about your struggles and aspirations not only promotes understanding but also deepens connections. This type of openness can build a foundation of trust and empathy, enabling those you care about to support you in the truest sense. For instance, sharing your fitness goals or sobriety milestones with friends invites their encouragement and help, which can be tremendously motivating.

Imagine having a support network that knows exactly what you're striving for; they can offer tailored advice or even a listening ear when times get tough. Clear communication helps identify areas where they can be helpful — whether it's joining you for a morning run, preparing healthy meals together, or simply offering words of encouragement. In this way, openness transforms passive observers into active participants in your sobriety and wellness journeys.

Engaging friends and loved ones in your fitness plans can further enhance motivation and consistency. When fitness becomes a shared goal, it adds a layer of accountability and motivation. You are more likely to stick to your routine when someone else is counting on you. Consider organizing regular activities like yoga sessions, hiking trips, or local sports matches. Doing so not only makes exercise enjoyable but also fosters a sense of team spirit and camaraderie, which can be vital for in the long-term.

Shared fitness ventures bring a little element of fun and variety to routines that could otherwise feel repetitive. It's less of a challenge to stick to a work-out routine when it's coupled with laughter, a little socializing, and friendly competition. Also working out with others can expose you to new activities, expand your interests and help make getting physically fit a fun part of almost every day.

Asking friends and family members to participate in physical activities together is not only beneficial to you but also be a catalyst for them and others around you. When involving friends in group workouts or pushing each other into reaching individual records, you help foster a supportive and nurturing environment. These types of initiatives do not just remove obstructions, but also blur the definitions of 'supporter' vs. 'participant,' spurring reciprocal encouragement towards healthier lifestyles for all involved. This common pursuit brings opportunities for discussion and finding similar interests and common ground.

Moreover, enlisting others makes for collaborative obstacles and achievements. The realization that a family member or friend has achieved a fitness goals or triumphed over a personal demon can motivate others to fully commit to their own health adventures. Taking time to acknowledge these for one another fosters a sense of community and helps instill a culture of encouragement and resilience.

Another great way to reinforce positive behaviors is helping your network celebrate progress. Public recognition of achievements—large and small—can be a powerful motivator. It reminds you of how much progress you've made, which is empowering and encourages you to keep going. Even if the celebrations are informal — an office party or a simple social media post — they can make these milestones more meaningful.

By sharing your successes, you're not only celebrating personal growth, but also inspiring those around you. You can inspire others to take steps of their own through a similar situation. This also serves to create a ripple effect by encouraging others to celebrate their wins and have a more positive approach to their struggles.

By sharing both the journey and the victories, it creates a feedback loop of motivation, where support generates success and success generates more support. It's not merely a conversation about results; it recognizes the work that it takes to get there. Through this practice, you shift the focus away from win-loss outcomes to process-oriented ones that emphasize perseverance and hard work.

Joining Support Groups

In the pursuit of healing and health, it may be all the difference to find a community that understands your struggles. Joining a support group is entering an environment where support and understanding are offered without reservation. The members of these groups have all walked a similar path; they understand the delicate balance of navigating personal challenges such as fitness or sobriety.

Imagine sitting in a room where everyone understands as you share your story—this is the power of engaging with those who relate to your struggles. Your challenges do not feel so insurmountable when met with collective understanding, and this connection fosters a profound sense of belonging. It's an affirmation that you're not alone and that others genuinely comprehend what you're going through. This is what many people have found in the rooms of Alcoholics Anonymous.

Alcoholics Anonymous groups serve not just as sources of emotional support but also as invaluable wells of strategies and perspectives, with each member contributing their unique experience to the collective wisdom. One person might share a helpful approach to staying sober during social events, while another offers insight on managing cravings or building a stronger support network. The diverse range of perspectives broadens your horizons and introduces new methods for navigating challenges on the path to recovery. AA groups provide exposure to different ways of achieving and maintaining sobriety, turning obstacles into powerful opportunities for growth and learning.

Moreover, many fitness groups have structured programs that incorporate activities designed to boost both physical and mental health. Such groups can serve as support groups for your fitness journey. This could be anything from organizing group workouts to holding meditative sessions aimed at stress reduction. Such activities are crucial because they instill discipline and consistency—two pillars essential in any recovery journey. Regularly participating in these activities helps build a routine, which is especially important for those committed to maintaining sobriety or improving fitness.

Participating actively in these programs also means you're expanding your social circle in a meaningful way. Within these circles, friendships form, morphing into lifelong support systems. The bonds created in such groups aren't merely based on shared interests but on a mutual commitment to wellness and encouragement. These relationships offer continuous support; even during tough times, there's always someone ready to lend an ear or provide guidance.

Creating accountability within these groups is another significant benefit. While it may not be necessary to outline strict guidelines here, the essence lies in how naturally accountability forms in such settings. Knowing that others are aware of your goals and progress can enhance motivation and ensure consistency. In many instances, the supportive push from peers keeps individuals on track toward achieving their health objectives.

Ultimately, joining a support group is not just about receiving help. It's also about giving back, sharing experiences, and building a network rooted in understanding, compassion, and mutual respect. As members of these groups, individuals contribute to a culture that reinforces positive change. In doing so, they help create an empowering environment where everyone feels encouraged and motivated to stay true to their recovery path.

Celebrating Progress and Milestones

Celebrating achievements is an essential component in fostering a supportive environment for those dedicated to fitness and sobriety. Recognizing milestones publicly not only builds confidence but also encourages continued progress. When individuals' efforts are acknowledged, it can reinforce their sense of accomplishment and motivate them to pursue further goals. This public acknowledgment acts as a powerful reminder that the journey they are on is valued by others too, thus deepening their commitment.

Imagine the power of hearing your name called out during a group meeting or seeing your achievement acknowledged in some public way. It demonstrates that your hard work has not gone unnoticed. It's more than just a momentary boost; it helps solidify internal motivation by connecting personal success with communal appreciation. As individuals are recognized, they feel validated and trusted within their community, which may encourage them to maintain these positive habits and push through challenging times.

Celebrations also play a crucial role in reinforcing positive behavior. They act as markers of hard work and perseverance. When a person reaches a milestone—like a month of sobriety or completing a fitness challenge—a celebration acknowledges this effort. It tells the person, "You've done well, and we're here to celebrate you." Such recognition does wonders for mental health, lifting spirits and reinforcing that the effort put into maintaining sobriety or enhancing fitness is worth it.

Everyone has times when motivation is low. Setbacks are part of any change process, and celebrations help offset these low periods by focusing on success instead of failure. By perpetually recognizing achievements, no matter how small, communities instill a habit of gratitude in individuals for their accomplishments, regardless of where they are on their journey. It's about creating a supportive narrative that highlights progress over perfection.

Furthermore, these celebrations encourage a culture of support and positivity in the members of a given community. If you celebrate the success of one, it is used to ignite inspiration/hopes for others who are still struggling for their goal. One success breeds hope, and people think in their own minds that they can work through whatever problems they have. This community-wide celebration bonds all taking part together, reminding that wins are shared, and completing a broader sense of community.

Involving family, friends, and peers in these celebrations can further cement this cultural shift towards positivity and shared success. It expands the circle of influence beyond immediate participants, involving those who care about their well-being. For instance, organizing a small gathering to commemorate someone's 1 year of sobriety can make a significant impact. Sharing in these moments reinforces bonds and fills the social spaces with encouragement and warmth.

Highlighting achievements not only supports those recognized but also serves as an inspiration to others. It promotes an uplifting environment for personal advancement and collective growth. When newcomers to a sobriety group or fitness class see the positive reception of others' successes, they understand that they have entered a place where progress is championed. This reassurance can ease fears, reduce feelings of isolation, and increase willingness to engage fully with the group's mission and activities.

Furthermore, sharing stories of accomplishments acts as a motivational tool for individuals at different stages of their journey. Whether someone is just beginning or has been working on their goals for years, there is always something to learn from others. Hearing firsthand accounts allows people to draw parallels between experiences and apply successful strategies to their own lives. It provides concrete proof that reaching milestones is possible, even amidst life's complexities.

Encouraging this type of environment also aligns well with modern psychological understandings of change and recovery. Positive reinforcement and community support are recognized drivers of personal transformation. Celebrating achievements taps into these principles, creating empowering scenarios that keep individuals engaged and hopeful. Knowing that their progress will be acknowledged and celebrated makes participants more likely to commit fully to both fitness and sobriety goals.

Reflecting on Supportive Environments

Building a network that embraces what we aspire for requires active involvement, where family and friends play an integral role. By sharing your goals and milestones with them, you create an environment rich in support and understanding. This openness transforms relationships, fostering shared experiences that reinforce commitments to healthy living. As loved ones become active participants, not just observers, they help maintain motivation and accountability. Activities like group workouts or meal planning become avenues for mutual encouragement, deepening bonds while collectively pursuing wellness. This cooperative effort goes beyond personal growth—it's about building a supportive community where everyone contributes to each other's success.

Continuing the path of recovery is greatly enhanced by joining a support group of individuals who truly understand your journey. Such communities provide safe spaces where empathy and shared experiences abound, reducing isolation. Diverse strategies and a collective wisdom pave the way for new approaches to health and well-being. Celebrating achievements within these circles further strengthens this communal bond, reinforcing positive change. When milestones are publicly acknowledged, it motivates continued progress and inspires others. This culture of celebration and encouragement acts as a driving force, ensuring that everyone remains committed to their sobriety and fitness journeys.

CHAPTER 11

Prioritizing Self-Care

G rowing up as the son of an alcoholic, I learned to navigate a world that felt constantly unstable. My father's drinking created chaos, and as a child, I often felt as if I needed to keep the peace. I became hyper-aware of his moods, always anticipating the next crisis and adjusting my behavior to avoid triggering his anger or despair. Without realizing it, I carried that sense of responsibility into adulthood, believing it was my job to fix everything and everyone around me. It wasn't until I began to confront my own alcoholism that I realized how deeply co-dependency had shaped me in my life.

When I first heard someone say "self-care is not selfish," it might as well have been in another language because I certainly didn't understand its meaning. For much of my life, my identity was tied to taking care of others, to the point where I didn't even know what my own wants and needs were anymore. Sobriety forced me to look in the mirror and reckon with the fact that I couldn't pour from an empty cup. If my cup was empty, then I had nothing to give someone else. I had to unlearn a lot of behaviors. I learned that taking care of myself wasn't just necessary for my own recovery—it was the best way to really show up authentically for other people. Slowly, I began to see self-care as something that paradoxically allowed me to better be there for others.

In my experience, prioritizing self-care plays a key role in maintaining sobriety and improving both physical and mental well-being. As individuals embark on a new life in sobriety, understanding the importance of self-care is vital. Self-care is not just about occasional indulgences or temporary escapes but involves cultivating habits that nurture the body, mind, and spirit consistently. In this chapter, we explore how integrating self-care into daily routines can help build a strong foundation for enduring sobriety and healthier living.

Throughout this chapter, we will explore effective strategies for incorporating self-care into busy lives without feeling overwhelmed. We will examine practical time management tips that ensure self-care remains a priority, even amid various responsibilities. Readers will also learn about setting healthy boundaries to protect their self-care practices. Additionally, we'll discuss the role of social support in building sustainable routines and identify how recognizing burnout signs can prompt timely adjustments in self-care strategies. By the end of the chapter, readers will have actionable insights to create personalized self-care plans that align with their unique needs on the road to sobriety.

Balancing Self-Care with Other Responsibilities

Before we get into the details of balancing self-care with the rest of your life, let's cover what "self-care" is and what it isn't.

When we fly on commercial flights, during the safety briefing conducted just before take-off, we hear about oxygen masks dropping down in the event of a loss of cabin pressure. We are instructed to secure our own masks before attempting to assist others. The rationale behind these instructions is that if we pass out from lack of oxygen, then we would be unable to be helpful to someone else. Similarly, if we prioritize our recovery from alcoholism, we set ourselves up to be better versions of ourselves in all other aspects of our lives. If we relapse, those better versions of us are unlikely to materialize. This is self-care and not selfish behavior.

On the flip side, I have seen people in recovery groups who keep themselves so busy doing various activities in and around recovery that they are never home and never have to face the wreckage their alcoholism has brought to their lives. In doing this, you'll always see them at recovery meetings but they never seem to have the time to do step work with a sponsor and they somehow manage to post-pone dealing with the consequences of their past actions. In effect, they have found a new method of escapism. This is not prioritizing recovery and is not self-care. In such an example, a person would be prioritizing distraction from life instead of recovery.

When someone prioritizes everything else in life over their own re-covery, they need to pause and look for an unbiased and honest assess-ment of their motivations. In my experience, the root of such lack of focus on recovery is often in fear—fear of judgment from others, fear of being perceived in some unfavorable light, or a need for external val-idation through positive affirmation when doing things to make others happy. On an individual-by-individual act basis this may seem altruis-tic—but, in actuality it is often quite self-centered and driven by an in-ternal focus to manage those fears or to seek the approval of others. Balancing recovery with life's demands requires recognizing that true self-care is not selfish—it's essential. Without it, the foundation of so-briety weakens, leaving both the individual and their loved ones at greater risk.

It's often easier to recognize in someone else when they are putting the wrong priorities on things in their lives. They may be ignoring re-covery or so immersed in recovery related activities as to avoid their lives. So how can we tell the difference in ourselves if we are putting the right priorities on things? This is an example of when a sponsor can be invalu-able because they can be more objective than we can be on ourselves. Besides the guidance of a sponsor, the key ingredient is balance. I have found that in every aspect of live when I am out of balance, it is at the expense of some other part of my life. So, I am always striving for bal-ance but even now—after years of walking this path—I still sometimes need the unbiased counsel of my sponsor.

At the beginning of our sobriety journey, finding balance and prac-ticing self-care can seem like a daunting task amid the chaos of our lives. Effective time management strategies play a crucial role in ensuring that self-care becomes an indispensable part of our routines. By utilizing tools like planners or digital calendars, individuals can visualize and allocate specific times for all the areas of life needing attention. This not only helps prioritize these moments but also ensures that some activities don't become overshadowed by other things. For instance, setting aside fifteen minutes every morning for meditation or a brief walk can lay the foundation for a more balanced day. In the early stages of sobriety, I kept a calendar where I scheduled my workday, workouts, recovery meetings, and my various life responsibilities. I tried to stay flexible and adjusted as needed—but, this calendar overview helped me to be more aware of what priorities I was assigning to things.

Establishing healthy boundaries is an important aspect of dedicating time to self-care without encroaching on other responsibilities. This might involve learning to say "no" to commitments that would overextend one's capacity or creating designated specific times within your schedule for various activities. Boundaries are not about excluding others but rather about protecting our well-being so that we can be present and functional in our roles as employees, friends, or family members. For example, consider communicating with family members that you have set aside an hour in the morning before work for the gym and an hour in the evening for recovery related activities. Involving family and friends in establishing this can be a great way to include them in the development of the schedule which helps reinforce their support of the plan and the healthy boundaries you're trying to establish.

When included in the development of our self-care routines, loved ones can also act as accountability partners. They can gently remind us of what we are trying to do when needed and help us stay engaged in a balanced way in all areas of our lives. Open dialogues about the importance of self-care in maintaining sobriety and our health can foster understanding and support from those around us. This collaborative approach enriches relationships and encourages shared activities like group exercises or cooking healthy meals together, which can enhance the overall experience.

Recognizing signs of burnout is critical in refocusing priorities towards self-care before reaching a breaking point. Common indicators such as constant fatigue, irritability, and a sense of detachment can signal the need for immediate attention to one's physical and mental needs. By acknowledging these signs early on, individuals can proactively adjust their self-care practices to prevent further decline. Whether it means scheduling a spa day or simply taking a day off work to relax and recharge, addressing burnout symptoms promptly is important and should be considered necessary for self-care.

Effective self-care stems from understanding that taking care of oneself is not a luxury but a necessity. It's crucial to view it as an integral part of daily life, alongside other commitments. Time management strategies can help ensure that self-care doesn't become an afterthought but remains a priority. Utilizing planners and calendars reminds you to dedicate time to yourself regularly, reinforcing the notion that self-care is just as important as any other appointment or obligation.

Boundary-setting empowers individuals to protect their self-care practices from being interrupted by external demands. It emphasizes the idea that saying "no" is as powerful as saying "yes" when it comes to maintaining balance. Creating clear limits around personal time is vital for preserving energy and focus, ultimately leading to more effective engagement in other areas of life.

Social support is a cornerstone in building a sustainable self-care routine. When family and friends understand and respect one's need for self-care, it creates a nurturing atmosphere where individuals feel encouraged rather than guilty for taking time for themselves. This underscores the idea of having loved ones involved in establishing what a balanced approach to recovery, fitness, and life looks like. Activities can also be shared, turning self-care into moments of joy and connection rather than solitary obligations. Consider taking a spouse to an open recovery meeting so that it is a shared experience or to the gym for a couple's workout.

Addressing burnout before it spirals out of control is necessary to staying on-track. Recognizing stressors and implementing strategies to mitigate them through proactive self-care can prevent severe consequences on health and sobriety. Building awareness around personal limits and responding to them with kindness and action promotes long-term benefits and resilience.

Flexibility in Self-Care

It's important to understand that adapting your self-care practices to fit into your current obligations doesn't make them any less impactful. In fact, the opposite is often true. Short, focused sessions of self-care can be just as effective as longer routines, enabling individuals to maintain their commitment without overwhelming their schedule. A brief ten-minute meditation each morning or a simple breathing exercise while commuting can offer profound benefits, setting a positive tone for the day. The key lies in emphasizing quality over quantity, ensuring that each session is meaningful and centered on personal growth.

Investigating adaptable self-care options that integrate seamlessly into everyday life is another powerful approach. Many may feel daunted by the idea of dedicating large blocks of time to self-care activities, particularly with the numerous roles they play daily—be it as a parent, employee, student, or partner. However, weaving self-care into routine tasks can help alleviate this pressure. For instance, opting to put in some ear buds and take a walk during a conference call not only provides physical exercise but also keeps us engaged in our responsibilities to others. Integrating these type of activities helps ensure that self-care becomes a natural part of one's lifestyle rather than an additional thing tacked onto the end of an already busy day.

It's equally essential to regularly evaluate the effectiveness of our self-care strategies. What worked at one stage of life might not hold the same benefits under different circumstances. Adopting a reflective approach allows individuals to assess whether their practices meet their current needs or if adjustments are necessary. Journaling can be a useful tool here, providing insights into emotional states and helping identify patterns over time. By keeping track of these reflections, it becomes easier to notice when changes in routines are required to maintain emotional and physical well-being.

Moreover, as life progresses through various stages, maintaining a flexible mindset is paramount for navigating challenges without compromising self-care. Changes such as business travel, starting a new job, moving to a different city, or even shifts in family dynamics can disrupt established routines. Yet, a willingness to adapt these routines can prevent feelings of being overwhelmed. Developing a toolkit of self-care practices that can be tailored according to changing circumstances ensures resilience and continuity. For instance, on particularly busy days, a ten-minute break to step outside and appreciate nature might suffice, whereas on quieter days, a longer meditation session could be more appropriate.

Adapting self-care practices to fit current obligations requires an understanding of one's own needs and the courage to adjust accordingly. This exploration becomes a personal journey of discovery, where finding what works best involves both experimentation and patience. Observe how your body and mind respond to different practices; this feedback is invaluable in tailoring a self-care plan that thrives amidst life's demands.

Some people struggle with the concept of personalized plans and believe that one-size-fits-all approaches work best. They do not see the value in a customized plan. However, an individualized approach acknowledges that each person's path in life may will look a little bit different—and that is okay. Embracing personalized strategies encourages autonomy and empowers individuals to make choices based on their preferences. Perhaps reading a chapter of a favorite book is more restorative for one person, while another might find solace in creating artwork.

Allowing oneself the freedom to choose inherently fosters a sense of self control and satisfaction.

Sustained Well-Being

Imagine a self-care plan as a roadmap to wellness. By setting clear objectives, you provide yourself with tangible milestones that can be both motivating and reassuring. These goals should be as unique as the person they serve. For instance, someone might aim to incorporate 15 minutes of mindfulness meditation daily or dedicate time to a hobby that brings joy and satisfaction. The key here is specificity, allowing for precise tracking. When you see progress, even in small increments, it reinforces positive behavior and provides encouragement to continue the path.

Integrating small, consistent self-care tasks into your daily routine is another fundamental aspect of a successful plan. Think of these tasks as building blocks; while each may seem small on its own, collectively, they form the foundation of lasting well-being. Consistency is crucial here. Simple activities like taking a short walk during lunch breaks, practicing gratitude journaling at night, or preparing a nutritious meal can have cumulative benefits. Over time, these practices become habits, naturally incorporated into the day, requiring less conscious effort and serving as daily reminders of your commitment to health and sobriety.

As life is dynamic, so too must be your self-care plan. Regularly reviewing and adjusting your strategy ensures it remains relevant and effective. Consider scheduling a weekly or monthly check-in with yourself to assess how well your plan aligns with your current needs and circumstances. Are there areas where you've grown and need new challenges? Or maybe certain parts of the plan no longer resonate or feel beneficial. Making adjustments keeps the process engaging and helps prevent stagnation.

Moreover, building resilience through adaptive self-care strategies is vital for long-term well-being. Resilience acts as a buffer against stressors and setbacks, proving invaluable when navigating the complexities of maintaining sobriety. Adaptive strategies could involve learning new coping skills, such as progressive muscle relaxation or cognitive-behavioral techniques, which can be applied in various situations. Resilience also flourishes when you're equipped to manage unexpected changes or challenges gracefully.

In addition to these steps, communicating needs effectively can foster a mutually supportive dynamic among loved ones. By expressing what you require in terms of support and understanding, you pave the way for relationships built on collaboration and empathy. Encouraging shared self-care practices can further strengthen these bonds. Whether it's participating in a fitness class together or organizing a weekly family dinner, shared activities create a sense of accountability and solidarity.

Equally important is seeking help and cooperation from others, which can significantly reduce feelings of isolation. Being open to accepting assistance not only lightens the load but also nurtures a network of support around you. Whether it's seeking advice from a mentor, attending group meetings, or simply confiding in a friend, these connections remind you that you're not alone in your pursuit of health and happiness.

Sustainable self-care goes beyond temporary fixes; it's about creating a lifestyle that fosters continuous growth and stability. For those committed to sobriety, embedding these principles into everyday life offers a pathway to thriving rather than merely surviving. It's about making informed, deliberate choices that honor your unique journey, with the understanding that self-care isn't a destination but a lifelong practice.

While acknowledging the transformative power of self-care, remember that it's a deeply personal endeavor. There are countless ways to nurture oneself, and experimentation may be necessary to find what resonates most meaningfully. Be patient, maintain flexibility, and above all, stay committed to prioritizing your well-being.

Reflecting on Self-Care

Understanding the necessity of self-care in maintaining health and sobriety is more than acknowledging its importance—it's about actively integrating it into everyday life. This chapter has explored how self-care, balanced with other responsibilities, becomes a cornerstone in nurturing both mental and physical health. By setting boundaries, creating routines, and utilizing time management tools, individuals can ensure that self-care doesn't fall by the wayside amidst daily demands. Engaging family and friends fosters a supportive environment that enhances these practices, transforming them into shared experiences rather than solitary tasks. Recognizing signs of burnout and addressing them promptly helps prevent setbacks and maintains holistic well-being.

For those newly embarking on their journey to sobriety or anyone seeking improved health, the message is clear: self-care isn't just an additional task but a vital, lifelong commitment. Flexibility in self-care practices allows for adaptation as life changes, ensuring personal needs are continually met. Regularly evaluating and adjusting self-care strategies keeps them relevant, empowering individuals to thrive rather than merely survive. The path to wellness requires patience and experimentation, recognizing that each person's approach will differ. By prioritizing self-care as an essential component of daily life, we lay a robust foundation to navigate life's challenges with resilience and strength.

CHAPTER 12

Conclusion

Choosing sobriety is a courageous step, one that opens doors to a healthier, more fulfilling life. Embracing this path means understanding the complex relationship between alcohol and your well-being. The detrimental impact alcohol has on both mental and physical health is undeniable, making it imperative to acknowledge these effects fully. When we ignore the risks associated with alcohol consumption, we risk facing grave consequences that can derail our lives.

The knowledge we've shared highlights why change is not just beneficial — it's necessary. Recognizing how alcohol can harm you mentally and physically is a start. This awareness serves as a wake-up call, urging us to address the root of the problem rather than just its symptoms. By identifying these issues, you are already demonstrating commitment to a better future where these harmful impacts no longer hold power over you.

In addition to acknowledging the adverse effects of alcohol, adopting positive lifestyle changes makes the recovery journey more manageable and sustainable. A key aspect of this transformation involves engaging in regular physical activity. Exercise acts as a cornerstone for improving mental clarity and emotional stability, both of which are essential during recovery. It's about more than just breaking a sweat or shedding a few pounds — it's about feeling accomplished and boosting your mood naturally. Regular workouts can also provide an effective coping mechanism, offering a productive outlet for stress and emotions rather than turning back to old habits.

Consider what happens when you integrate something like yoga into your routine, combining it with meditation practices. These mindfulness exercises offer profound benefits. They do more than just help you relax; they empower you. With enhanced self-awareness and emotional regulation, you are better equipped to confront and manage potential triggers. Moreover, by cultivating a clearer mindset through mindfulness, you drastically reduce the likelihood of relapse. This strategic approach ensures that your mind and body work together harmoniously, supporting you every step of the way.

Another pivotal element in nurturing your health is establishing a sustainable nutrition plan. Your body needs the right fuel to heal and thrive, especially after the toll alcohol has taken. Eating balanced meals supports not only your physical health but also influences your emotional state and resilience. By investing time in understanding your nutritional needs, you unlock another layer of healing. Just as a car cannot function without the correct fuel, your body cannot operate at its best without proper nourishment.

Every effort you make towards maintaining a balanced diet directly contributes to your overall well-being, creating a stable foundation from which you can draw strength during challenging times. It's amazing how much of our mental and emotional health links back to the foods we eat. Proper nutrition enhances mood stability and cognitive functions, providing you with yet another tool in your recovery arsenal.

While it's important to implement these changes, remember that patience and perseverance are vital. Sobriety is not a destination but a continuing journey. Some days will be tougher than others, but with the strategies and knowledge gained from this book, you are better prepared to face them. Lean on the community surrounding you — friends, family, support groups. Their encouragement and shared experiences can be invaluable. You are never alone in this process. Countless individuals have walked a similar path and emerged stronger, proving that recovery is indeed possible.

Your commitment to sobriety extends beyond personal benefits and impacts those around you in profound ways. By choosing to live a healthier life, you inspire others who may still be struggling to see that change is achievable. You become a beacon of hope, showing the world the power of determination and resilience. Your journey can ignite change in others, creating a supportive network that thrives on shared victories and lessons learned.

Keep in mind progress is a journey. Acknowledge every milestone, no matter how small; any sober day is a win. Strive to nourish and nurture the relationships which now can be much healthier and holistic now that alcohol no longer has the louse grip on your life. It takes incredible strength and courage to choose this route, highlighting how much you want to grow as a person and build a life of happiness.

Final thoughts, trust in your ability to build a better tomorrow. Know that each positive decision brings you nearer to who you are becoming. There is so much to explore, and this is your journey to own. Embrace this new chapter with conviction and the knowledge and tools to succeed. Your journey will not always be easy, but it will be rewarding, one that will bring you a life characterized by true joy, peace, and fulfillment.

Bonus Material

The Twelve Step Guide and Workbook by Josh Grant. Available on Amazon in Kindle, Paperback, and Hardcover. The audiobook is also available through Audible. This workbook is designed to be used by someone going through the Twelve Steps of Alcoholics Anonymous with a sponsor. Inside you will find guidance and reading assignments along with suggestions. The physical copies of the book provide insightful and probing questions as well as all of the Twelve Step Worksheets. The Kindle and Audiobook versions present the same material with instructions to write the answers separately.

The book may be found on Amazon and Audible at the following links:

English	https://www.amazon.com/dp/B0DP3DXXZF
Spanish	https://www.amazon.com/dp/B0DQF6HQ1B
Audiobook	https://www.amazon.com/Twelve-Step-Guide-Recovery-Alcoholism/dp/B0DS2W91N2/

The first 50 people to send an email requesting a discount code to **Info@Recovery4Life.US** will receive access to a free version of The Twelve Step Guide available through Audible.com

www.ingramcontent.com/pod-product-compliance
Lightning Source LLC
Chambersburg PA
CBHW060941120626
46557CB00003B/1089